Soft Tissue Injuries in Sports Medicine

Soft Tissue Injuries in Sports Medicine

edited by

Louis C. Almekinders, MD
Associate Professor
Division of Orthopaedic Surgery
Sports Medicine Section
University of North Carolina at Chapel Hill School of Medicine
Chapel Hill, North Carolina

**Blackwell
Science**

Blackwell Science

EDITORIAL OFFICES:

238 Main Street, Cambridge, Massachusetts 02142, USA

Osney Mead, Oxford OX2 0EL, England

25 John Street, London WC1N 2BL, England

23 Ainslie Place, Edinburgh EH3 6AJ, Scotland

54 University Street, Carlton, Victoria 3053, Australia

Arnette Blackwell SA, 1 rue de Lille, 75007 Paris, France

Blackwell Wissenschafts-Verlag GmbH
  Kurfürstendamm 57, 10707 Berlin, Germany
  Feldgasse 13, A-1238 Vienna, Austria

DISTRIBUTORS:

North America
Blackwell Science, Inc.
238 Main Street
Cambridge, Massachusetts 02142
(Telephone orders: 800-215-1000 or 617-876-7000)

Australia
Blackwell Science, Pty. Ltd.
54 University Street
Carlton, Victoria 3053
(Telephone orders: 03-347-0300 fax: 03-349-3016)

Outside North America and Australia
Blackwell Science, Ltd.
c/o Marston Book Services, Ltd.
P.O. Box 87
Oxford OX2 0DT
England
(Telephone orders: 44-1865-791155)

Acquisitions: Michael Snider
Development: Debra Lance
Production: Paula Card Higginson
Manufacturing: Kathleen Grimes
Printed and bound by Edwards Brothers, Ann Arbor, MI

Library of Congress Cataloging-in-Publication Data
Soft tissue injuries in sports medicine / [edited by]
  Louis C. Almekinders.
    p. cm.
  Includes bibliographical references and index.
    ISBN 0-86542-382-2
    1. Soft tissue injuries. 2. Sports injuries.
  I. Almekinders, Louis.
    [DNLM: 1. Athletic Injuries. 2. Soft Tissue
  Injuries.   QT 261 S681 1996]
  RD97.S638 1996
  617.1'027—dc20
  DNLM/DLC
  for Library of Congress   95–36197
                                                        CIP

To Sally

Contents

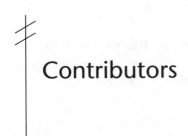

Contributors

Louis C. Almekinders, MD
Associate Professor of Orthopaedic Surgery, Sports Medicine
Section, University of North Carolina at Chapel Hill School of
Medicine, Chapel Hill, North Carolina

Eugene E. Berg, MD
Associate Professor of Orthopaedic Surgery, University of South
Carolina School of Medicine, Columbia, South Carolina

William L. Craig III, MD
Division of Orthopaedic Surgery, University of North Carolina
Hospitals, Chapel Hill, North Carolina

Walton W. Curl, MD
Associate Professor of Orthopaedic Surgery, Bowman Gray School
of Medicine; Director, Sports Medicine Unit, Wake Forest
University, Winston-Salem, North Carolina

Lisa T. DeGnore, MD
Assistant Professor of Orthopaedic Surgery, University of Kentucky
College of Medicine, Lexington, Kentucky

Charles J. Gatt, MD
Fellow, Orthopaedic Sports Medicine, Department of Orthopaedic
Surgery, Cleveland Clinic Foundation, Cleveland, Ohio

D. Montgomery Hunter, MD
Department of Orthopaedics, Department of Emergency Medicine,
Bowman Gray School of Medicine, Sports Medicine Unit, Wake
Forest University, Winston-Salem, North Carolina

Uffe Jørgensen, MD, PhD
Associate Professor, Section of Sports Traumatology, University of
Copenhagen; Chief of Sports Medicine Copenhagen County,
Gentofte Hospital, Copenhagen, Denmark

Eugene L. Kastelberg, Jr., MD
Associate Professor of Sports Medicine and Family Medicine, Department of Orthopaedics, Virginia Commonwealth University, Medical College of Virginia, Richmond, Virginia

David F. Martin, MD
Assistant Professor of Orthopaedic Surgery, Bowman Gray School of Medicine, Sports Medicine Unit, Wake Forest University; Guilford College of Sports Medicine, Winston-Salem, North Carolina

Richard D. Parker, MD
Staff Physician, Department of Orthopaedic Surgery, Cleveland Clinic Foundation, Cleveland, Ohio

William E. Prentice, PhD, PT, AT, C
Professor and Coordinator of Sports Medicine and Specialization, Department of Physical Education, Exercise, and Sport Science; Clinical Professor of Physical Therapy, Department of Medical Allied Health Professions; Associate Professor of Orthopaedics, The University of North Carolina at Chapel Hill School of Medicine, Chapel Hill, North Carolina; Director, Sports Medicine Education and Fellowship Program, HEALTHSOUTH Rehabilitation Corporation, Birmingham, Alabama

Lisa R. Reznick, MD
Hand Fellow, Department of Orthopaedic/Plastic Surgery, University of Rochester School of Medicine and Dentistry, Rochester, New York

Bryan W. Smith, MD, PhD, FAAP
Clinical Assistant Professor of Pediatrics and Orthopaedics, University of North Carolina at Chapel Hill School of Medicine; Head Team Physician, James A. Taylor Student Health Service, University of North Carolina at Chapel Hill, Chapel Hill, North Carolina

Timothy N. Taft, MD
Max M. Novich Professor and Director of Sports Medicine, University of North Carolina at Chapel Hill School of Medicine, Chapel Hill, North Carolina

O.E. Tillman, MD
Sports Medicine Fellow, University of North Carolina at Chapel Hill School of Medicine, Chapel Hill, North Carolina

Preface

In the past decade, there has been an enormous increase in the number of health professionals interested in the treatment of sports injuries. This has resulted in a vast amount of sports injury research in the pathophysiologic, diagnostic, and therapeutic aspects of these injuries. This increasing interest and knowledge has brought about significant changes in the diagnosis and treatment of injured athletes. Initially these changes were evident in the early, aggressive, invasive treatment of fractures with internal fixation of the injuries. This approach often minimizes the athlete's time away from practice and competition, it can avoid the deconditioning effects of prolonged immobilization, and allows accurate restoration of the injured structures. Research on soft tissue injuries has lagged behind that on the treatment of fractures, but during the last several years similar approaches have emerged in the treatment of ligament, muscle, and tendon injuries. Research has shown that many soft tissue injuries are better treated with early, aggressive, mobilization techniques. Traditional approaches such as prolonged casting, withdrawal from any type of sports for an entire season, and other "wait and see" attitudes have not been shown to stimulate the healing process or even to be detrimental. An active approach with early mobilization has shown excellent results in many soft tissue injuries. Often, improved functional results are obtained much sooner than by using more traditional approaches. Occasionally, surgical treatment is needed to make early mobilization possible.

However, soft tissue injuries are not only seen and evaluated by surgeons but also by primary care physicians, physical therapists, athletic trainers, coaches, and even fellow athletes and parents. *Soft Tissue Injuries in Sports Medicine* is aimed at those readers who did not receive formal training in the treatment of sports injuries. The first part covers the basic principles of anatomy, physiology, response to injury, and treatment. A basic understanding of these principles is needed for the second part, which discusses the most common sports injuries by anatomic area. Soft tissue injuries comprise the vast majority of all musculoskeletal sports injuries. In addition, most soft tissue injuries are minor, and can be easily diagnosed and treated by health professionals at the primary care level. This book allows the reader to recognize minor injuries. Major injuries that will need to be referred to sports medicine specialists are discussed only to allow recognition and appropriate handling prior to referral. The book incorporates the latest knowledge on sports injuries as it is relevant for the primary care health professional. Finally, it is meant to be a source of information for involved coaches, concerned parents, and injured athletes themselves.

Louis C. Almekinders

Acknowledgment

I am grateful to Ms. Dana Hedgepeth for her editorial and secretarial assistance in the production of this book.

PART ONE

Basic Principles

CHAPTER 1

The Anatomy, Histology, and Biochemistry of Soft Tissue

Louis C. Almekinders

Excellence in the care of musculoskeletal injuries begins with a clear understanding of the relevant basic sciences. Clinical practice must be guided by knowledge of the normal structure and function, the mechanism of injury, and the characteristics of the normal healing process. Without this knowledge the care of injured athletes will be based on pure chance and luck. Greater knowledge in basic sciences has led to significant improvements in the injury care provided by those practicing sports medicine, which in the past often was based solely on tradition and custom. This chapter will cover the basic macroscopic, microscopic, and biochemical aspects of soft tissues in the musculoskeletal system.

Ligaments and Tendons

Ligaments and tendons are flexible, strong fibrous bands that provide stability and allow muscles to exert their actions. They are discussed together because they share many common anatomic and biochemical features.

Ligaments are connections between two bones and are generally found around joints. By connecting the two bones within or outside the joint capsule, they often provide the majority of the stability for the joint. The joint is designed to allow a certain range and direction of motion. Ligaments will restrict abnormal motion in directions for which the joint was not designed. Ligaments can also restrict excessive motion in the joint's normal plane of motion. Ligaments can be found both outside and inside the joint. Inside the joint they are always covered with a thin layer of tissue, the synovial lining. Outside the joint ligaments either are thickened bands within the joint capsule or actually are completely separate from the capsule that surrounds the joint (Fig. 1.1).

Tendons are connections between muscles and bones (Fig. 1.2). Therefore the tendons allow the muscles to move the bone when the muscle contracts and shortens. Virtually all muscles are connected to bone through a tendon. The length of the tendon, however, is highly variable. Sometimes tendons can be many inches long, but occasionally they are only several millimeters long. Tendons like those in the hand and foot need a large amount of excursion and move over a relatively large area. Large excursion is needed because toes and fingers need to move over a large distance. Such tendons develop specialized sheaths around them that improve the gliding properties of the tendon. These synovial sheaths have a lining that has many

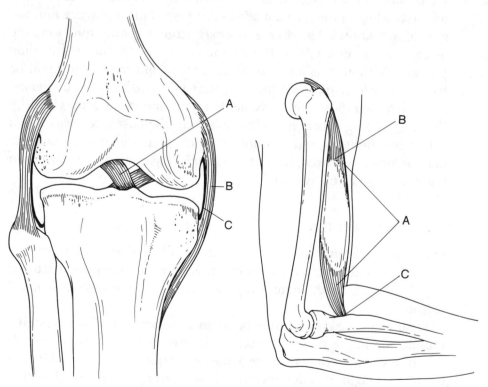

Figure 1.1 *Ligaments both inside (A) and outside (B) the joint capsule (C).*

Figure 1.2 *A muscle-tendon unit with the tendon (A) connected to the muscle (B) and the bone (C).*

properties similar to those of joint lining—in particular, the production of a fluid that acts as a lubricant.

The ground substance that lends ligaments and tendons their strength is a protein called collagen. The collagen molecule is a long spiral that forms strong crosslinks with other collagen molecules (Fig. 1.3). Numerous collagen molecules are laid down in parallel fashion and form small tendon or ligament fibers. A group of ligament or tendon fibers makes up an entire ligament or tendon. This arrangement gives ligaments and tendons excellent strength when placed under tensile forces. Small, flattened cells called fibrocytes or fibroblasts live interspersed between the collagen bundles (Fig. 1.4). The cells have an active metabolism and maintain the surrounding collagen matrix.

Both ligaments and tendons have a well-defined blood supply. Small blood vessels penetrate the tendons and ligaments and provide

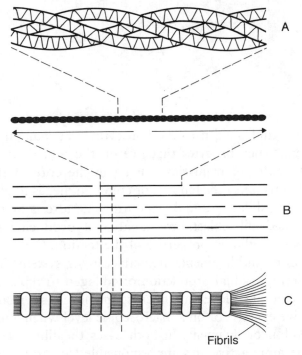

Fibrils

Figure 1.3 *Crosslinked collagen molecules (A) joined together into fibrils (B) eventually form a ligament or tendon (C).* (Redrawn by permission from Martinez-Hernandez A, Amenta P. Basic concepts in wound healing. In: Leadbetter WB, Buckwalter JA, eds. Sports-induced inflammation. Park Ridge, IL: American Academy of Orthopaedic Surgeons, 1990:57.)

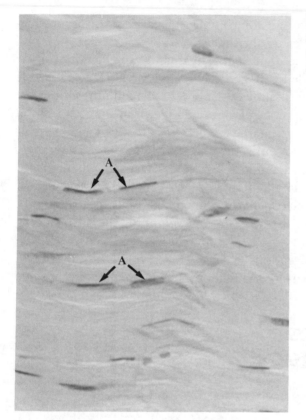

Figure 1.4 *Photomicrograph of a tendon showing fibroblasts or fibrocytes (A) living between the collagen bundles.*

nutrients and oxygen to the fibrocytes that maintain the tendon or ligament. The fibrocytes that live on the outside of the tendon are slightly different from those living in the core of the tendon. The outside surface of the tendon, or epitenon, needs to glide smoothly as the tendon slides up and down during and after a muscle contraction. The outside fibroblasts are capable of producing substances that improve the gliding properties of the tendon.

Tendons and ligaments are active, living systems in which there is a constant, gradual production of collagen to replace injured tissue. Injury can take place on a microscopic level as a result of strenuous, repetitive exercise or on a macroscopic level when a major force tears the tendon or ligament. In both cases the fibrocytes or fibroblasts become more active and are responsible for producing new collagen to heal the defect. There are small biomechanical differences between ligaments and tendons. These differences are mainly in the type of collagen molecules that are produced, the size of collagen bundles, and the degree of metabolic activity.

The collagen fibers assume a wave-type pattern if the tendon or ligament is not under stretch (Fig. 1.5). The wave pattern or crimp disappears if the structure is placed under sufficient tension. This is accompanied by a slight elongation of the tendon or ligament. The elongation is usually no more than 2% to 4% of its original resting length. Stretching the ligament or tendon beyond that point would injure the collagen. Removal of the force that led to the straightening of the crimp pattern will result in return to the resting length with reappearance of the crimp.

Both ligaments and tendons have connections with the central nervous system. Through these connections messages from receptors within the tendon or ligament are relayed to the central nervous system. This provides the brain with information regarding the tension and position of the involved structure. The ability to provide constant information regarding the position of our body and its extremities in space is termed proprioception. Research has shown that patients with a chronically torn ligament in or around a joint have a decreased sense of position of the involved joint. This impaired proprioception has also been associated with an increased likelihood of degenerative arthritis within that joint.

The attachment site of ligaments or tendons to bone is a highly specialized area (Fig. 1.6). The collagen fibers of the ligaments or tendons are generally deeply anchored within the bone. These specialized fibers are often called Sharpey's fibers. In addition to fibers anchoring into the bone, there are fibers that are continuous with the membrane covering the bone, the periosteum, adding to the strength of the attachment site. Occasionally the transition between tendon and bone contains a small zone of cartilage (see Fig. 1.6).

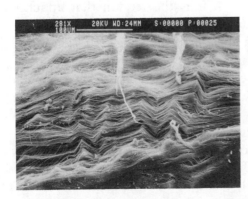

Figure 1.5 *Scanning electronmicrograph showing the wave pattern or crimp of the collagen fibrils in tendon.*

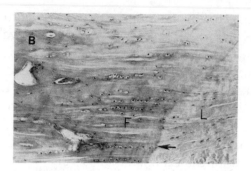

Figure 1.6 *Photomicrograph of a ligament-bone junction. The ligament (L) attaches to the bone (B) through a zone of fibrocartilage.* (Reproduced by permission from Woo SL-Y, Gomez MA, Sites TY, et al. The biomechanical and morphological changes in the medial collateral ligament of the rabbit after immobilization and remobilization. J Bone Joint Surg 1987;69A:1207.)

Muscle

Muscles can be activated to bring about motion through contractions. They are also continuously active to maintain the body's posture, position, and stability. Generally muscles are never without tension, and their resting tone adds to the stability of most joints. Continuous active contraction during walking and standing is necessary in many antigravity muscles to maintain posture. Without the stabilizing action of muscles, the spine would collapse and the joints would give way during any upright activity. In addition to their stabilizing action, they are capable of moving and accelerating parts of the body or the entire body. The vast majority of muscles act on the bones of the spine and extremities.

The attachment of the muscle is generally through tendons. The muscle belly attaches to the tendon at the musculotendinous junction on each side of the belly (Fig. 1.7). It is the tendon that attaches to the bone (see section above on ligaments and tendons). The musculotendinous junction is a highly specialized area (Fig. 1.8). Collagen fibers from the tendon are actually anchored into the ends of the muscle fibers. The entire musculotendinous junction often extends over a large part of the muscle. Sometimes it extends along two thirds of the side of the muscle belly (see Fig. 1.7). This is thought to distribute the stress over a larger area.

When the muscle contracts it often moves the two attachment sites of the muscle closer together. The change between these points of origin and insertion of the muscle and its tendon is called the excur-

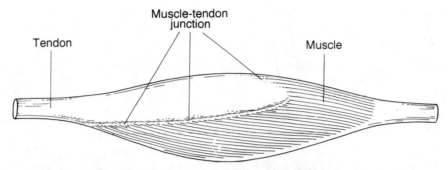

Figure 1.7 *Muscle, tendon, and muscle-tendon junction.*

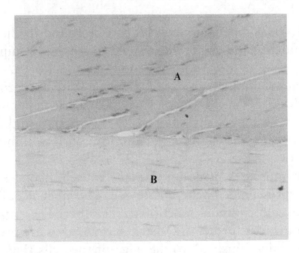

Figure 1.8 *Photomicrograph of a muscle-tendon junction. The muscle fibers (A) attach to the tendon (B) in an oblique manner.*

sion of the muscle. When the musculotendinous junction extends along a large part of the muscle belly, the muscle fibers are relatively short. They also attach at a higher angle to the tendon than do muscles with a short musculotendinous junction (Fig. 1.9). This results in a muscle that has a large cross-sectional area and therefore is strong. However, the excursion of such muscles is relatively short. Strength with little excursion are characteristics generally found in antigravity muscles that maintain posture such as the muscles around the spine. Larger excursion and less strength are found in the muscles of the forearm and lower leg that control the fingers and toes.

Grossly, muscles have either a single muscle belly (unipennate) or multiple bellies that converge into a single tendon (multipennate)

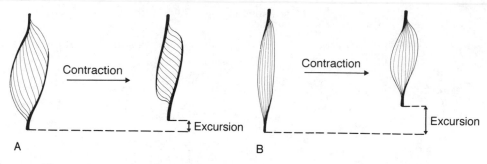

Figure 1.9 *A muscle with a long muscle-tendon junction and short excursion (A) and a muscle with a short muscle-tendon junction and long excursion (B).*

(Fig. 1.10). Unipennate muscles can be found in the forearm where they function as finger flexors or extensors. Unipennate muscles usually have a short musculotendinous junction and with large excursion and limited strength are better suited to provide fine motor skills. Multipennate muscles, such as the gastrocnemius muscle in the calf, have a longer musculotendinous junction and are more suited for providing strength and stability with a limited amount of excursion.

Each muscle is made up of many muscle fibers. Each fiber essentially represents a single muscle cell. The fiber usually extends from one musculotendinous junction to the other. The muscle fiber is filled with contractile proteins. Other cell organelles are present as well but are generally "pushed" to the edge of the cells (Fig. 1.11). Multiple nuclei, mitochondria, and other organelles can be found in every muscle cell. All the muscle fibers are being held together by connective tissue. This connective tissue is divided in epimysium, perimysium, and endomysium. As individual, skinned muscle fibers without con-

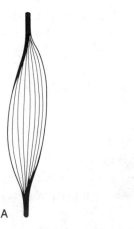
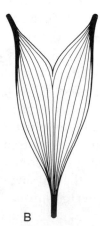

Figure 1.10 *A unipennate muscle (A) and a multipennate muscle (B).*

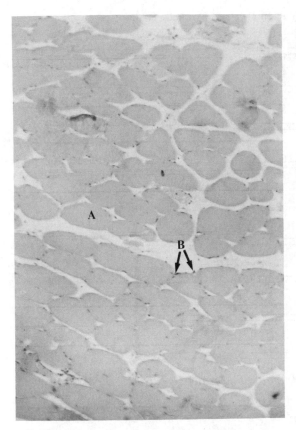

Figure 1.11 *Photomicrograph of a cross section of skeletal muscle. Each fiber is filled with contractile proteins (A), and the multiple nuclei (B) are near the outside of each fiber.*

nective tissue can easily be stretched without resistance up to two or three times their original length, this connective tissue serves an important role in preserving the integrity of all fibers within one muscle. It lends the entire muscle some stiffness and resistance to stretch and allows the muscle to work more efficiently. Each muscle has a rich blood supply. Blood vessels often enter the muscle both along with the nerve that supplies it as well as in other separate locations. Smaller blood vessels or capillaries reach the individual muscle fibers along the connective tissue network of the perimysium and endomysium.

The biochemical components that give the muscle its unique capability to contract actively are the contractile proteins. Large protein molecules within the muscle cell, such as actin and myosin, can actively engage and generate a contracting force (Fig. 1.12). The active engagement of these protein filaments is initiated when a nerve impulse arrives at the muscle cell and releases calcium into the cell. The calcium is normally stored outside the muscle cell but "leaks" through the cell membrane when a nerve impulse arrives in the

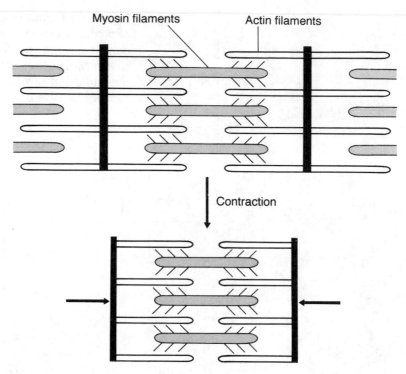

Figure 1.12 *Contraction through engagement of actin and myosin components in muscle.*

muscle. The increased calcium concentration within the cell allows a number of chemical events to occur that lead to contraction of the muscle fiber.

The active engagement of the muscle proteins costs energy. Some energy is readily available and stored within the muscle fiber. However, this generally is only sufficient for a few seconds of active contraction of the muscle. More energy will have to be generated for exercise that lasts beyond this. The muscle can do this through various pathways. The two main pathways are a relatively quick one without the use of oxygen and a slower pathway that allows the use of oxygen.

The quicker pathway, called glycolysis, allows quick but still short bursts of activity. The glycolytic pathway is quick but relatively inefficient. In return for energy it yields a waste product, lactate. Lactate is an acid and can quickly accumulate and interfere with muscle activity, leading to fatigue and decreased strength. Glycolysis is therefore mainly used by the muscle for short events like sprinting or weight lifting. Longer events, in particular endurance sports, cannot rely on the quick but relatively inefficient glycolysis.

Another pathway, termed oxidative phosphorylation, is slower to respond but yields significantly more energy. Furthermore, it is not associated with poorly tolerated waste products such as lactate. Rather, it results in the production of carbon dioxide and water, which are easily disposed of through the lungs and kidneys. One of the main limiting factors for this pathway is the availability of oxygen, which is needed to convert the fuel into energy. Training will minimize this limitation by improving lung function, oxygen-carrying potential of the blood, and oxygen delivery to the muscle.

Not all muscle fibers are the same. First, there is a distinct difference between muscles that one can voluntarily control and those one cannot control. Involuntary muscle is found in intestines and around blood vessels and many other internal organs. Involuntary muscle cells do not have any clear markings when viewed under a microscope and are therefore termed smooth muscle cells. In contrast, in voluntary muscle cells the contractile proteins are arranged in a very distinct pattern. This results in the typical striation seen under the microscope (Fig. 1.13). Voluntary muscle is therefore often called

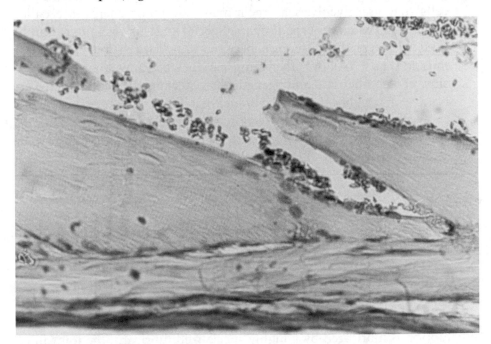

Figure 1.13 *Photomicrograph of two muscle fibers near the muscle-tendon junction. Cross-striation in the fibers is visible under this high-power magnification.*

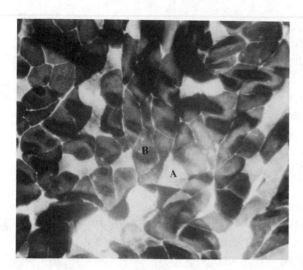

Figure 1.14 *Photmicrograph of a muscle with a special histochemical stain that shows slow twitch fibers (light-colored, A) and fast twitch fibers (dark-colored, B).*

striated muscle. Within striated muscle a distinction can be made on the basis of which energy pathway is most commonly used in that particular muscle cell. Muscle cells that use predominatly oxidative phosphorylation are called red, slow twitch, or type I fibers. Muscle cells that use glycolysis as their main source of energy are called white, fast twitch, or type II fibers. Special staining techniques can be used to reveal the difference between slow twitch and fast twitch muscle (Fig. 1.14). Whether a muscle fiber becomes a fast twitch or slow twitch fiber is mainly genetically determined. Some athletes are born with a higher percentage of fast twitch fibers and are more likely to excel in events that require only short bursts of energy. Training can improve the efficiency of existing fibers but does not appear to be able to permanently change one fiber type to another.

Cartilage

Cartilage is not truly a soft tissue but is also different from a hard tissue like bone. Most cartilage is found in the joints, where it can be seen as two different types. Hyaline or articular cartilage is the white, glistening cartilage that covers the ends of the bones within the joint (Fig. 1.15). As the joint moves, the articular cartilage portions slide past one another and result in a painless, smooth movement. This motion is lubricated by a highly specialized lubricant, the joint fluid. It is produced by specialized cells in the joint lining and contains special macromolecules that lend the fluid its lubricating properties. No synthetically made lubricant has yet to even approach the lubricating qualities of joint fluid. In some joints like the knee and the shoulder, the joint surfaces do not perfectly fit together. Some of the voids on the edge of such joints are filled up by separate pieces of cartilage (see Fig. 1.15). This cartilage is structurally different from hyaline cartilage and is called fibrocartilage.

Cartilage is a unique structure because most of it lives without any direct blood supply. Cartilage cells receive their nutrition from joint fluid, which carries the nutrients to the edge of the cartilage. By a process of diffusion the nutrients slowly move through the cartilage. The cells that live within the cartilage are called chondrocytes. Similar to the fibrocytes, they actively maintain the substance or matrix around them. One of the important ground substances of cartilage matrix is collagen. Unlike tendons and ligaments, the collagen in cartilage is generally arranged in arcades rather than parallel bundles (Fig. 1.16). In this way articular cartilage is better able to withstand compressive forces, which is one of its crucial functions. The space around the collagen bundles is also filled with a highly specialized ground substance. Proteoglycans are molecules that are produced by chondrocytes by linking proteins and sugars together. This results in a large molecule that is able to attract and hold water molecules very well. The result is a stiff but at the same time somewhat spongy tissue that is very well designed to absorb loads occurring during physical

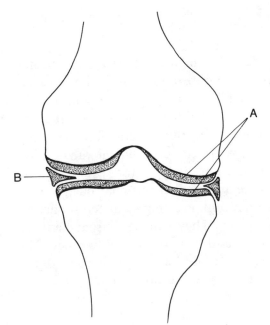

Figure 1.15 *Hyaline cartilage (A) and fibrocartilage (B) in a knee joint.*

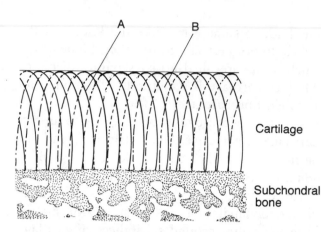

Figure 1.16 *Collagen fiber arrangement (A) and location of proteoglycans (B) in articular cartilage.*

Cartilage

Subchondral bone

activity such as running and jumping. Through this shock absorption it protects the underlying bone and at the same time allows smooth motion to occur in the joint.

Fibrocartilage is somewhat different from hyaline cartilage. It contains not only collagen fibers but also a significant number of elastin fibers. The fibers are oriented in a more parallel fashion, which renders the cartilage more resistant to tensile loads. The fibrocartilage in the shoulder and knee is still important to disperse compressive loads. On the other hand, fibrocartilage is also attached to soft tissue, which exerts tensile loads on the structure as well.

Bursa

In areas where different structures have to slide past one another during activity, friction occurs. To minimize friction the body develops a bursa. It is usually a thin sac filled with a small amount of fluid (Fig. 1.17). The fluid acts similarly to joint fluid and lubricates the walls of the bursa. During motion the fluid-filled bursa virtually eliminates the friction between the two structures. Bursae can develop anywhere in the body that friction occurs—for example, the prepatellar bursa around the knee and the subacromial bursa above the shoulder. Other bursae can develop in response to certain activities required during sports activities. They can be present between moving tendons, underneath skin, and near bony prominences. The cells that line the wall of a bursa are somewhat similar to some of the cells found in the lining of a joint. They are responsible for producing the fluid within the bursa.

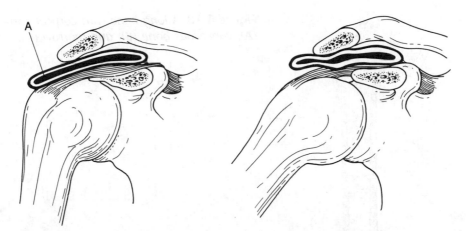

Figure 1.17 *A bursa (A) around the shoulder that minimizes friction between the moving parts.*

Bone

This section will briefly discuss the structure of bone in order to give a complete understanding of all the components of the musculoskeletal system. Soft tissues often attach to bony structures, and knowledge regarding the structure of bone can be helpful in understanding and diagnosing soft tissue injuries. Two types of bone are found in the skeletal system. Cortical or compact bone is the dense bone that makes up the shaft of most of our long bones. Cancellous bone is much more porous bone and is found predominantly in small bones and at the ends of long bones (Fig. 1.18). All bone is maintained by living cells or osteocytes. In compact bone they live within the bone supplied by small blood vessels that travel through tiny canals within the bone. In cancellous bone the osteocytes live both within and on the surface of the bone. The blood supply of cancellous bone is much more abundant because of the porosity of the bone, which allows more and larger blood vessels to penetrate it. The ground substance of bone again begins with collagen molecules. However, after the collagen is produced by the cells, calcium salts are laid down on top of the collagen bundles. This results in the mineralization of bone and its hard structure.

The outside of the bone is covered by a thin layer called the periosteum. It harbors cells that are capable of duplication and pro-

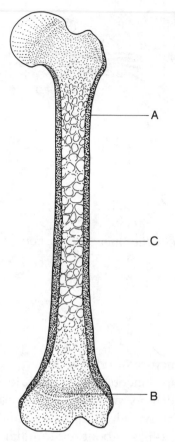

Figure 1.18 *A long bone with cortical bone (A), cancellous bone (B), and marrow (C).*

duction of more bone in cases of injury such as fractures. Inside the bone, marrow can be found. The primary function of marrow is the production of blood cells, but it also harbors cells capable of repairing bone.

Nerve

For the body and the extremities to move, one needs to send messages to the muscles to tell them what to do. On the other hand, the brain needs to receive messages back that give information regarding the speed, position, contact with other surfaces, and encounters with painful stimuli. With this information the brain can give the muscles messages to adjust the movement by stopping, accelerating, or making it more efficient. This neuromuscular control is accomplished by motor and sensory nerves and becomes better in athletes as a result of training.

Motor nerves have their cell body in the central nervous system or spinal cord and relay the impulses through long tentacles called axons to the muscles (Fig. 1.19). Axons can therefore be several feet long in order to reach the muscles in the extremities. Each axon is surrounded by a myelin sheath. This fatty-like substance is produced by Schwann cells that live between the axons, within the nerve itself. The myelin sheath improves the electrical properties on the axon and allows the electrical impulse to be propagated more efficiently along the axon. Each motor axon supplies several muscle fibers. The group of muscle fibers and their supplying motor nerve is called the motor unit (see Fig. 1.19). In areas where fine control over each muscle is needed, such as the finger flexors, there are relatively few muscle fibers in each

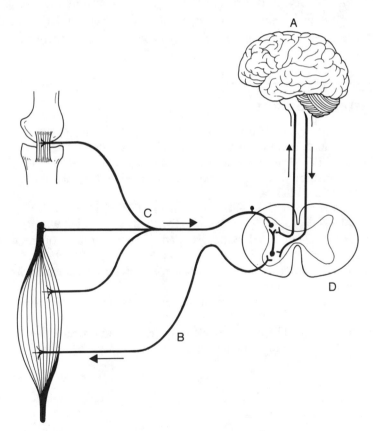

Figure 1.19 *Central and peripheral nervous system. The brain (A) sends impulses through motor nerves (B) to the muscles. It also receives sensory information from ligaments, muscles, and tendons (C). The spinal cord (D) serves as a relay station.*

motor unit. In muscles that are used mainly for power, such as the muscles around the spine, there are many more muscle fibers in each motor unit.

The sensory input is picked up by sensory nerves that may have their cell body outside the central nervous system. Many different kinds of sensory nerves have been identified. Pressure-sensing nerve endings are particularly common in the skin whereas tension-sensing nerve endings are more often seen in muscles, tendons, and ligaments. As the sensory nerve endings relay information regarding changes in pressure, tension, and position, the brain and spinal cord make adjustments through the motor nerves, often at a subconscious level. When no active, conscious thought process is needed to accomplish this, it is generally called a reflex. Many reflexes do not even require brain activity and are therefore termed spinal reflexes. The knee or ankle jerk seen following a quick stretch of the quardriceps or gastrocnemius-soleus muscle is an example of a spinal reflex.

Suggested Readings

Amiel D, Frank C, Harwood T, et al. Tendons and ligaments: a morphological and biochemical comparison. J Orthop Res 1984;1:257–265.

Gollnick PD, Armstrong RB, Saubert CW, et al. Enzyme activity and fiber composition in skeletal muscle of untrained and trained men. J Appl Physiol 1972;33:312–319.

Netter FH. The CIBA collection of medical illustrations, vol. 8: Part I. Musculoskeletal system. West Caldwell, NJ: CIBA-Geigy, 1990.

Owen R, Goodfellow J, Bullough P, eds. Scientific foundations of orthopaedics and traumatology. Philadelphia: WB Saunders, 1984.

Simon SR, ed. Orthopaedic basic science. Rosemont, IL: American Academy of Orthopaedic Surgeons, 1994.

Teitz CC, ed. Scientific foundations of sports medicine. Toronto: BC Decker, 1989.

Wilson FC, ed. The musculoskeletal system: basic processes and disorders. 2nd ed. Philadelphia: JB Lippincott, 1983.

CHAPTER 2

The Biomechanics of Soft Tissue Injury

Louis C. Almekinders

During normal daily activities the musculoskeletal system is continually subjected to mechanical stress. In an otherwise healthy person these stresses normally do not lead to injury. During sports activities the mechanical stress changes dramatically. This can be change in magnitude, direction, or duration of the stress. Each change alone or in combination can clearly lead to a breakdown in the musculoskeletal system. Many features of the injury that results can often be predicted if the magnitude, direction, and duration of the mechanical stress are know. Therefore knowledge of the biomechanical principles is important in understanding soft tissue injuries. Understanding the mechanism of injury also can help one determine how the injury should be treated and rehabilitated. It allows a more causal rather than empiric treatment. Finally, it can be important in prevention of the same or similar injuries both for the individual athlete and for other athletes involved in the same sports activity.

Biomechanical Principles

To understand the biomechanical literature it is important to understand the correct definitions of commonly used terms. Forces can be exerted on the body by placing an external load upon the body. The impact of another player during a collision is a common example of an external load. Other external loads are less obvious but can be equally important. Landing on the ground with a foot during the running motion also creates an external force. If the ground would not "push back" onto the foot, it would sink into the ground. However, normally the ground reaction force is an external force that prevents this (Fig. 2.1). In addition to external forces, many internal forces are generated. For the joint to remain stable during running and jumping, muscles need to contract actively. Active contraction is needed not only for propulsion but also for deceleration and shock absorption. This leads to the generation of internal forces. When all the internal and external forces are taken into account, many ligaments, tendons, and muscles have to withstand forces that exceed two or three times the body weight of the individual.

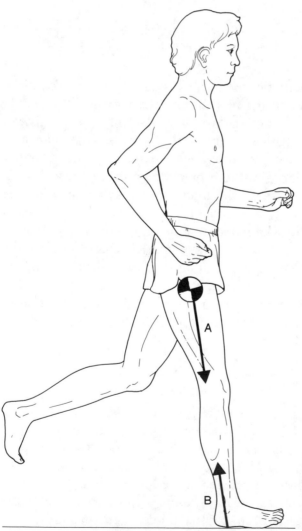

Figure 2.1 *The force due to body weight (A) and the resulting ground-reaction force (B) during heel strike of the running motion.*

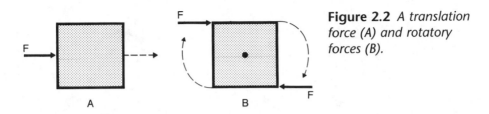

Figure 2.2 *A translation force (A) and rotatory forces (B).*

When an internal or external force or load is placed upon the body or a body part, it can result in motion if it is not balanced by other opposing forces. In biomechanical terms, two types of motion can result. It can be translation if there is one resulting force that acts in the direction of the translation (Fig. 2.2). Rotation will result if there are two resulting, parallel opposing forces that act upon the body in different places (see Fig. 2.2). In the body, motions are usually very complex and consist of both translation and rotation.

When a force is placed upon a body or body part and it is opposed by equal forces, no motion will occur. However, the body or body part will experience these forces as movement is being resisted. Three types of forces can be described in this situation. If the opposing forces point toward each other, they are called compressive forces. If they point away from each other, they are tensile forces. Finally, if they are opposing rotatory forces, they are called shear forces (Fig. 2.3).

Several anatomic terms are usually employed to describe joint or extremity position and motion (Fig. 2.4). First of all, the front of the body is called anterior, and the back is posterior. The top is termed superior or cranial, whereas the bottom is inferior or caudal. Medial is used for the inside (toward the midline), and lateral for the outside (away from the midline). Flexion and extension is a rotatory movement from posterior to anterior and back, respectively. Internal or

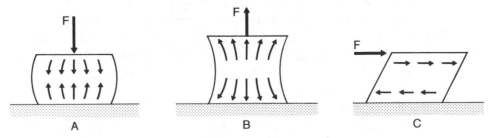

Figure 2.3 *A compressive force (A), tensile force (B), and shear force (C).*

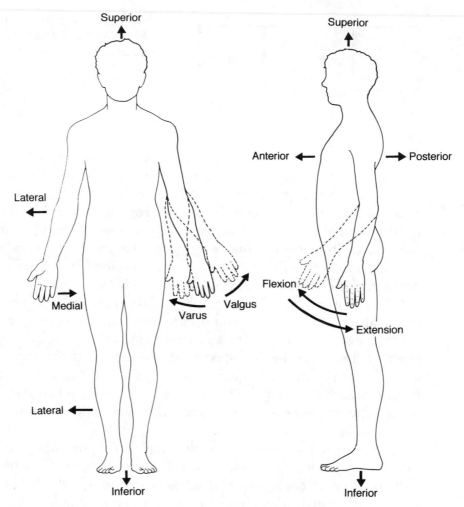

Figure 2.4 *Anatomic descriptions of position and motion.*

medial rotation is the description of a rotatory movement of the most distal body part involved toward the midline of the body. External or lateral rotation describes the opposite motion. Valgus or abduction describes an angulation or translation of the most distal body part involved away from the midline. Varus or adduction is the opposite, with motion toward the midline. Finally, translation can also be described by its direction, such as anterior or medial translation.

In order to standardize forces or load and make them comparable to other situations, they are often expressed as stress. The standardization is often done by calculating the force per unit. For instance, this unit can be the surface over which the force is exerted. In this manner it does not matter whether the person involved in the measurement was small or large, and the number can be compared with other measurements.

One of the unique features of the response of soft tissue to mechanical forces is its ability to deform. Any significant deformation without damage virtually does not occur in bone or other materials such as metals. Compressive, tensile, and shear forces all will initially result in deformation of muscle, tendon, ligament, and to a lesser extent cartilage. These structures are said to have viscoelastic behavior. The degree of deformation can be measured through the change of length or volume. Similar to the standardization of force or load to stress, the deformation can be standardized to strain. This is done by calculating the deformation per unit. The unit is usually the original length or volume.

By plotting the stress against the strain in a graph, a stress-strain curve is obtained that describes the viscoelastic behavior of a certain material (Fig. 2.5). If the deforming forces are not excessive, the deformation will stop at a certain degree, and if the forces are removed, the structure will regain its original shape without any evidence of damage or injury. Deformation without injury is termed elastic deformation and represents the first linear part of the stress-strain curve. An example of elastic deformation is stretching of a tendon until the crimp pattern is straightened. Release of the stretching forces will result in the return of the crimp pattern. If the deforming forces become too large, injury will occur to the structure. This will become clear when the forces are removed and the structure does

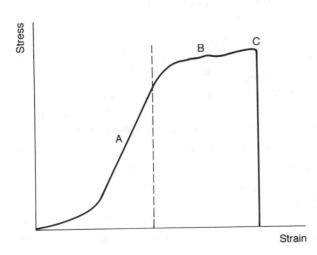

Figure 2.5 *Typical stress-strain curve of soft tissue. Increasing stress results initially in elastic deformation (A), followed by plastic deformation (B), and eventually failure (C).*

not return to its original shape. This is called plastic deformation. If the forces continue to increase, eventually complete failure will occur such as a rupture of the ligament. The ultimate yield point has been reached at that point. This will release the effects of the deforming forces, and the stress will return to zero.

Acute Soft Tissue Injuries

In most acute injuries the involved tissue is essentially normal just before the injury. External forces such as collisions and falls are responsible for the majority of acute injuries. The following section describes the biomechanical features of most acute soft tissue injuries.

Acute Ligament Tears

As discussed in Chapter 1 the ligaments provide much of the stability of the joint. While doing so they are mainly subjected to stretching or tensile forces. As the joint is moved into an abnormal or excessive range of motion, the ligaments restrain this motion as they are pulled taut. What constitutes abnormal or excessive motion is entirely joint-specific. In principle, four types of anatomic motion planes are possible. These are flexion-extension, internal-external rotation, translation, and abduction-adduction. Abduction and adduction can be similar to valgus and varus motion. Any significant amount of translation is usually an abnormal motion in most joints. Flexion-extension is generally the only normal motion in hinge joints, whereas rotation and abduction-adduction are also possible in ball-and-socket joints.

In most joints there are multiple ligaments that each have a primary function in restraining abnormal motion. Usually, each ligament is ideally suited to restrain one, sometimes two directions of abnormal motion. For instance, the primary stabilizer in the knee for forward movement (anterior translation) of the tibia on the femur is the anterior cruciate ligament. The anterior cruciate ligament also provides some stability to valgus forces if the medial collateral ligament (the primary stabilizer against valgus force) is already torn (Fig. 2.6). The anterior cruciate is therefore considered one of the secondary stabilizers against a valgus force.

Ligaments can stretch a certain amount without sustaining any injury. This elastic deformation is usually no more than 5% to 10% of its original length. If this amount is exceeded, the ligament is permanently injured owing to plastic deformation (see above, section

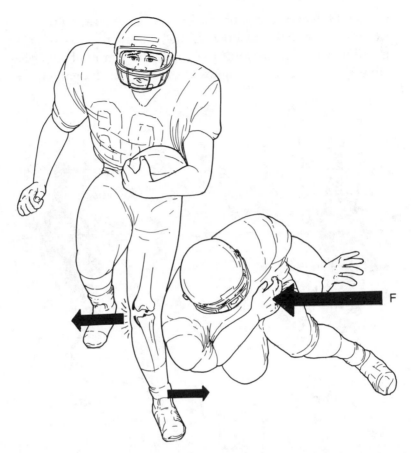

Figure 2.6 *Valgus-directed force (F) that results in medial collateral and anterior cruciate ligament injury.*

on biomechanical principles). Whether plastic deformation takes place is dependent on a number of factors. The magnitude of the offending force and the strength of the ligament are obvious factors that can determine the degree of injury. One of the less obvious factors is the speed with which the force is applied. If a force stretches the ligament relatively slowly, the ligament can often absorb more energy before it fails. Conversely, when a ligament is stretched more quickly, it can be more "brittle" and fail with less energy absorption. The strength of the ligament is not a constant factor either. On the one hand, aging and immobilization significantly weaken the ligament, in particular where it attaches to the bone. On the other hand, regular exercise can result in significantly stronger ligaments.

If the ligament is just barely stretched into the plastic region, virtually no instability of the joint will be detected on clinical examination. However, the patient will experience pain on the clinical stress examination of the ligament. This examination is done by putting manual stress on the joint that pulls the ligament taut (Fig. 2.7). In clinical terms this is diagnosed as a grade I ligament tear. If the

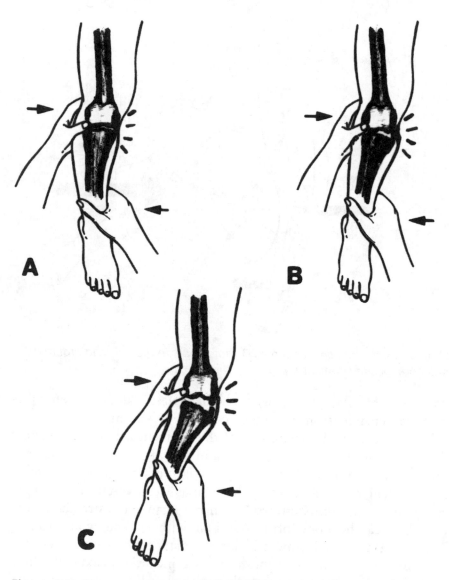

Figure 2.7 *Stress examination of the medial collateral ligament of the knee joint. Pain but no instability (A) signifies a grade I tear. Pain with some instability but a good endpoint (B) indicates a grade II tear, whereas absence of an endpoint (C) indicates a grade III tear.*

ligament was stretched well into the plastic deformation region but not to the ultimate yield point, a certain amount of instability will be noticeable on physical stress examination. However, eventually the remainder of the ligament will become taut and result in the presence of an "endpoint." This is diagnosed as a grade II ligament tear. If the yield point was exceeded at the time of injury, no endpoint will be present. This is a grade III ligament tear. On examination a grade III tear will feel as if there is nothing restraining the knee when one attempts to stress the involved ligament. Determining the grade of the ligament injury generally has important implications for the prognosis and treatment of the injured ligament. Specific stress examinations for each joint will be discussed in Part Two of this book.

Acute Tendon Injuries

Tendons have biomechanical behavior similar to that of ligaments. The contracting muscles will mainly result in stretching or tensile forces exerted on the tendons. Normally, muscle forces will result in stretching of the tendons that remains well within the elastic region. Only a small amount of stretch will occur in the region. If too much stretch were to occur, the muscle could not efficiently move the joints. It would dissipate the muscle forces into the stretch of the tendons. Ruptures of normal tendons are very uncommon because normal muscle forces are unable to stretch the well-designed tendons into the plastic deformation region. Therefore special circumstances are needed to cause a rupture of the tendon. The most common circumstance is a preexisting weakness of the tendon. Chronic tendinitis can weaken the tendon to such a degree that a sudden muscle contraction can rupture it.

A simultaneous antagonistic force can also contribute to the development of a tendon injury. This can occur if, for instance, an opponent forcibly flexes the knee as the quadriceps is trying to extend it (Fig. 2.8). The antagonistic force can also be an internal force from opposing muscle groups. It is thought that opposing muscle groups can suddenly overwhelm a contracting muscle and result in an injury.

An acute tendon injury tends to be an "all-or-none" phenomenon. Only complete tears will be obvious because of the absence of the muscle action through that tendon. Partial tears such as grade I and II tendon tears can be difficult, if not impossible, to diagnose.

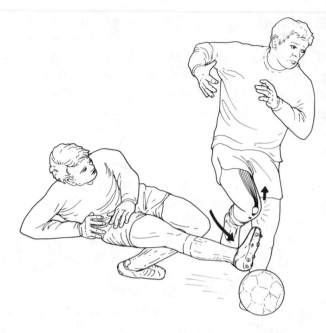

Figure 2.8 *A potential mechanism of injury resulting in a patellar tendon rupture. The quadriceps actively extends the knee but is forced into flexion by the opposing player.*

Acute Muscle Tears

When a muscle contracts it generates a certain amount of internal tension. The amount of tension that is generated is determined by the degree to which the muscle is stretched (Fig. 2.9). If the muscle is very shortened or lengthened, it cannot generate much contractile force. At its resting or neutral length, it can generate maximal tension or contractile force. Stretching beyond this point results in a drop of contractile force but also increases passive tension owing to stretching of the connective tissue framework of the muscle. Continued stretching will therefore result in increasing total tension within the muscle. Continued stretching will eventually rupture the muscle.

Injuries such as muscle rupture can occur if the muscle contracts and is stretched simultaneously. Stretching can be brought about by opposing antagonistic muscles (Fig. 2.10). Similarly to tendon injuries the forces can also be increased if the muscle is simultaneously stretched by an external force such as an opposing player or the ground-reaction force during a fall. These forces may be sufficient to cause a permanent plastic deformation of the muscle. It has been shown that these injuries take place in a very specific area of the muscle. The musculotendinous junction is by far the most common area where injury due to plastic deformation occurs (Fig. 2.11). It is

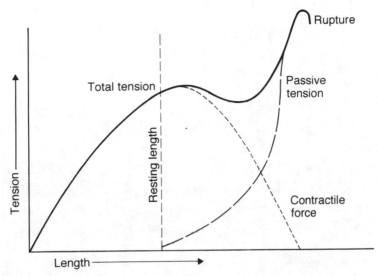

Figure 2.9 *The length-tension relation of skeletal muscle.* (Redrawn by permission from VanderWiel CJ, Hooker CW. Histology and biochemistry of muscle. In: Wilson FC, ed. The musculoskeletal system: basic processes and disorders, 2nd ed. Philadelphia: JB Lippincott, 1975:183.)

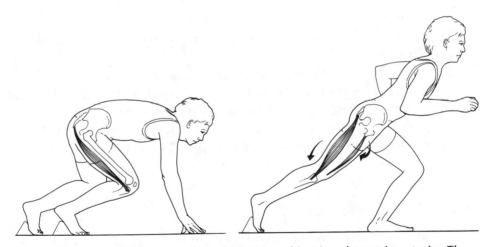

Figure 2.10 *Potential mechanism of injury resulting in a hamstring strain. The hamstrings actively contract to extend the hip but are stretched simultaneously due to knee extension.*

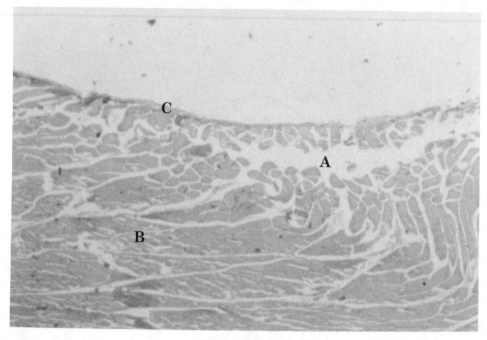

Figure 2.11 *Photomicrograph of an acute muscle tear. The tear (A) commonly occurs next to the junction of the muscle tissue (B) and the tendon (C).*

not entirely clear why the area is the weakest link of the muscle-tendon unit.

Tears of the muscle are divided into three grades similar to ligament injuries. A grade I tear signifies an injury that is associated with only a minor stretch of the muscle but without gross disruption. A grade II tear is a partial rupture of the muscle, whereas a grade III indicates a complete rupture of the muscle. Only in grade III tears is muscle action completely absent.

Chronic Soft Tissue Injuries

Relatively little is known about the biomechanics involved in the development of a chronic soft tissue injury. It appears that there are at least several ways for chronic injuries to develop. First, it is possible that the injury occurs as an acute injury. Inadequate treatment, poor healing conditions, or inadequate rehabilitation can lead to incomplete healing with resulting chronic pain and disability.

Second, chronic injuries can develop as the result of repetitive loading of a structure that eventually leads to an insidious, generally chronic injury. Each load by itself is not enough to injure the structure, but because of the repetitive nature of the load, eventually a "fatigue crack" occurs. Continued presence of the repetitive motion or load results in gradual accumulation of these microinjuries, which can lead to a chronic injury. A diagnosis of overuse injury, repetitive strain injury, or repetitive motion injury is often used in these situations.

Finally, it appears that some chronic injuries are related to intrinsic, often age-related changes. Aging is often associated with a weakening and slight stiffening of soft tissues. Mechanical stresses that are normally well tolerated in athletes in their twenties may lead to gradual tissue breakdown in older, poorly conditioned athletes. Many chronic soft tissue injuries have characteristics of all three components. It is important for the treating health professional to decide which factor plays the most important role in order to provide a rational treatment plan.

Chronic Ligament Injuries

Most ligaments are capable of handling repetitive low loads without any evidence of injury. Especially in the lower extremity the strength of the ligaments easily exceeds the stresses caused by repetitive motion such as running or jumping. In the upper extremity this is not always the case. In throwing athletes such as baseball pitchers or football quarterbacks, the repetitive throwing motion can cause gradual injury to the ligament. In particular, the ligaments of the shoulder and elbow are susceptible in these athletes (Fig. 2.12). It is not exactly clear how the injury occurs, but it results in a gradual stretching of the ligaments, usually without frank rupture. This results in instability of the affected joint.

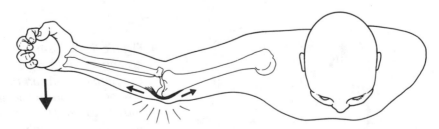

Figure 2.12 *The repetitive throwing motion can lead to a gradual stretching injury of the ligaments around the elbow.*

Chronic Tendon Injuries

Chronic injuries of tendon are extremely common in sports medicine. Tendons of both the upper and lower extremity can be affected. There appear to be two types of chronic tendon injuries. First, tendons can be injured by chronic friction of the tendon over a relatively prominent or rough area. This can be an external cause such as badly fitting athletic equipment (e.g., shoes, pads, or gloves). Internal causes such as a prominent bone or other tendon can also contribute to the problem. The repetitive and excessive friction generally cause an inflammation of the tendon sheath and is therefore often called tendinitis or paratenonitis.

A second form of chronic tendon injury is an injury caused by repetitive and excessive tension within the tendon. This usually occurs during eccentric contraction of the muscles. During an eccentric muscle contraction the muscle develops active tension but at the same time is forcibly lengthened. Such contraction is needed while the athlete is decelerating such as landing from a jump (Fig. 2.13) or during and after the heel strike of the running motion. Extremely high tension is generated within the muscle and its tendon during these eccentric contractions. This can result in a gradual breakdown of the tendon if the tendon is not trained enough to withstand this repetitive

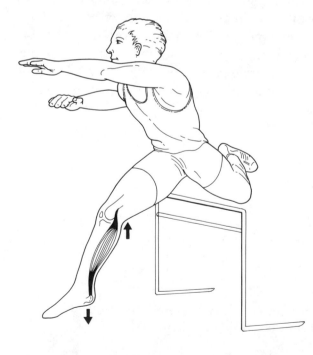

Figure 2.13 *Example of eccentric muscle action. As the hurdler lands on the forefoot, the gastrocnemius muscle contracts to dampen the impact but is also lengthened to allow the heel to come down to the ground.*

stress. The breakdown often occurs within the substance of the tendon near its insertion into the bone. Aging of the tendon often seems to make it more susceptible to this injury. Inflammation is not usually seen during this injury, and therefore it should be called tendinosis and not tendinitis.

Chronic Muscle Injuries

Relatively little is known about chronic muscle injuries. Chronic muscle pain is not uncommon and is often diagnosed as a chronic strain. Whether the muscle tissue is truly injured in these chronic strains is not clear. It is possible that other tissues such as the connective tissue of the muscle or scar tissue is actually responsible for the pain. Two types of subacute muscle injuries have been conclusively identified.

First, there appears to be a form of chronic compartment syndrome that can result in muscle pain. Most muscles in the extremities are grouped together in compartments. Each compartment is surrounded by an inextensible envelope, also called fascia (Fig. 2.14). During

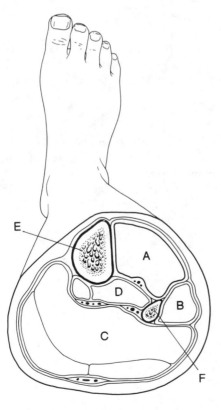

Figure 2.14 *The fascial compartments of the lower leg. The anterior (A), lateral (B), superficial posterior (C), and deep posterior (D) compartments are surrounded by a well-developed fascia and the tibia (E) and fibula (F).*

vigorous exercise the muscles swell because of the increase in the circulation. In addition, the muscle becomes gradually larger with repeated exercise as a result of a physiologic strengthening response. Occasionally the fascial envelope is too tight to allow this enlargement. The pressure during exercise increases within the compartment, which subsequently impairs the circulation through the compartment. The muscle may not receive enough oxygen and nutrients, which results in pain.

Another form of subacute injury is eccentric loading-induced muscle injury. Repeated eccentric contractions in a relatively untrained muscle can cause injury to the muscle on a microscopic level in the muscle fibers. Eccentric contractions are needed in many activities but are particularly forceful in activities such as downhill running. These muscle contractions are needed to dampen the impact and slow down the accelerating body. The muscle injury due to these eccentric contractions is often not obvious until 24 or 48 hours after the activity, when delayed onset muscle soreness manifests.

Suggested Readings

Armstrong RB. Mechanisms of exercise-induced delayed onset muscle soreness: a brief review. Med Sci Sports Exerc 1984;16:529–538.

Brewer BJ. Mechanism of injury to the musculotendinous unit. Instr Course Lect 1960;17:354–358.

Mow VC, Hayes WE, eds. Basic orthopaedic biomechanics. New York: Raven Press, 1991.

Noyes FR, DeLuccas MS, Tovik PY. Biomechanics of anterior cruciate ligament failure: an analysis of strain rate sensitivity and mechanism of failure in primates. J Bone Joint Surg 1974;56A:236–253.

Tipton CM, Matthes RD, Maynard JA, Carey RA. The influence of physical exercise on ligaments and tendons. Med Sci Sports 1975;7:165–176.

Viidik A. Biomechanical behavior of soft connective tissues. In: Akkas N, ed. Progress in biomechanics. Amsterdam: Sijfhoff and Noorthoff, 1979:75–113.

CHAPTER 3

The Response to Injury

Louis C. Almekinders

Chapters 1 and 2 review the basic anatomic and biochemical features of soft tissue as well as the biomechanical events leading up to injury of these tissues. Once an injury of the soft tissue occurs, a response will be generated by the local tissues and the remainder of the body in an attempt to heal the injury. This chapter will discuss the response of each tissue to acute or chronic injury. Soft tissues appear to be capable of responding to injury in a way that is common to all tissues, both hard and soft.

Many basic features can be seen in the response to injury throughout the body. However, each type of soft tissue has a different function, and in order to restore that specific function there are also distinct differences in the healing process between different types of soft tissue. A clear understanding of the common and specific features of the response to injury is needed to develop a rational treatment and rehabilitation plan for the injury. The treatment plan should be aimed at minimizing any inappropriate responses to the injury and maximizing responses that lead to rapid and functional recovery of the injury.

Acute Ligament Injuries

Most acute ligament injuries are ruptures caused by failure in tension as described in Chapter 2. The majority of the ligaments run outside the joint and are not in direct contact with the joint cavity. The first stage of the response to rupture of such ligaments is a classic inflammatory response. At the time of injury there is bleeding or hemorrhage into the area of the rupture. The athlete will notice a rapid onset of pain and swelling. The injury and the bleeding lead to the death, called necrosis, of cells such as the fibroblasts in the torn ends of the ligament. Ruptured collagen fibers are also present in this area.

The initial event liberates many substances from injured cells that evoke a cascading response from the remainder of the body (Fig. 3.1). These mediators of inflammation attract inflammatory cells that are normally circulating within the vascular system in a quiescent state. Inflammatory cells that can participate in this response are leukocytes, lymphocytes, and macrophages. Once attracted to the area of injury, they have numerous functions (see Fig. 3.1). One of the initial functions is to amplify the local response. The inflammatory cells will release additional mediators of inflammation that will cause more swelling or edema and attract more inflammatory cells. Many different mediators of inflammation have been identified. They include kinins, prostaglandins, leukotrienes, and complement factors. In addition to inflammatory mediators, other substances such as interleukins and tumor necrosis factor are released, and they can have adverse effects on other cells in the area. These substances, called cytokines, appear to play a role in every inflammatory response but

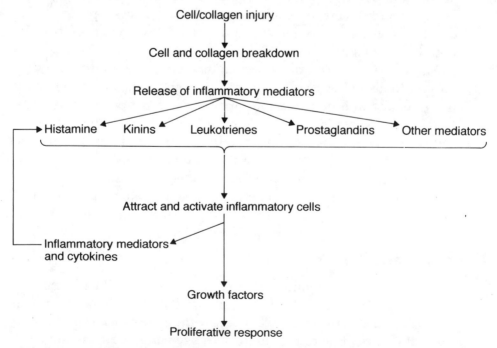

Figure 3.1 *The inflammation response following an acute soft tissue injury.*

their significance is not yet entirely clear. After 48 to 72 hours the entire area of the rupture is filled with inflammatory cells. The athlete will still experience significant pain and swelling, and initial stiffness is developing.

Another crucial function of the inflammatory cells is the initiation of a healing response. Healing seemingly can occur only after the dead cells and ruptured fibers have been cleared from the area of injury. Inflammatory cells are also needed for this function. In particular, the macrophage is a very efficient cell in cleaning up this debris.

Finally, the inflammatory cells are also capable of releasing factors that allow transition from the inflammatory phase of the injury response to the next phase, the proliferative phase. These substances, often called growth factors, are capable of stimulating growth in other healthy cells surrounding the injury. Stimulation of fibroblasts by these factors can cause them to migrate into the injured area and proliferate at the same time. Once the fibroblasts are present in the injured area of the ligament, they start producing new collagen. This new collagen will ultimately restore the mechanical function of the ligament by "mending" the two torn ends of the ligament together. Blood vessels or endothelial cells are also stimulated to grow and form new blood vessels that grow into the injured area. This provides nutrients to the proliferating fibroblasts. Gradually the inflammatory cells will disappear during this phase.

The final phase is the remodeling or maturation phase. The initial collagen that was laid down to repair the ruptured ligament is generally slightly disorganized and of less strength than the original ligament (Fig. 3.2). After several days to weeks of proliferation and production of collagen, the fibroblasts will remodel the injury site with more organized collagen bundles. The crosslinking of the collagen bundles will also increase, thereby increasing the mechanical strength of the healed ligament. After several weeks the ligament generally returns to its resting state. Even though the injury response is efficient, it often does not return the ligament to an entirely normal state. The ligament tissue at the healed site can be of slightly inferior quality. This can also be associated with residual laxity in the ligament. Treatment of ligament ruptures is generally aimed at diminishing the ill effects of the initial inflammatory phase and stimulating the proliferative and maturation phase. This is done by protecting the ligament from excessive stress during the initial healing phases in order to avoid residual laxity. Later during the healing controlled stress is placed on the partially healed ligament to stimulate matura-

3 days

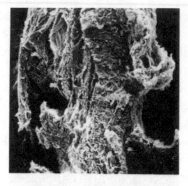

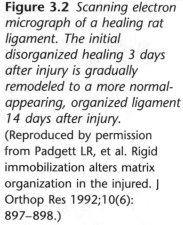

Figure 3.2 *Scanning electron micrograph of a healing rat ligament. The initial disorganized healing 3 days after injury is gradually remodeled to a more normal-appearing, organized ligament 14 days after injury.* (Reproduced by permission from Padgett LR, et al. Rigid immobilization alters matrix organization in the injured. J Orthop Res 1992;10(6): 897–898.)

7 days

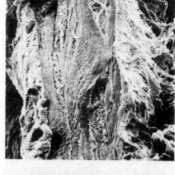

14 days

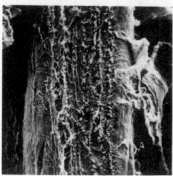

tion and remodeling. Chapter 4 will discuss the general treatment guidelines for these injuries.

The healing response of ruptured ligaments that run within the joint space appears to be quite different. Common examples of such ligaments are the cruciate ligaments of the knee. They are completely surrounded by joint fluid. The previously described phases are not as clearly present in these ligaments. In addition, the healing response often does not lead to a healed ligament (Fig. 3.3). Rather, the torn ends gradually round off and fail to attach to one another. It is not

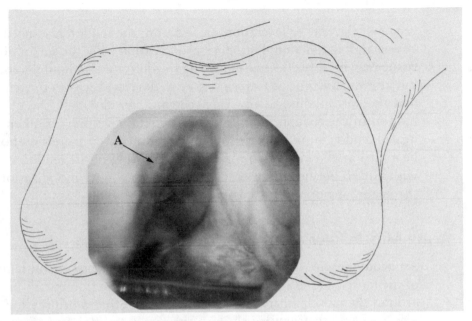

Figure 3.3 *Arthroscopic view of a knee 2 years after an anterior cruciate ligament tear. The injured ligament failed to heal and was largely resorbed leaving an empty intercondylar notch (A).*

entirely clear why this happens, but it is possible that the joint fluid that is present in these cases prevents a good healing response.

Acute Tendon Injuries

Many tendon injuries are caused by direct laceration with a sharp object. Occasionally a tendon can rupture indirectly from excessive tension within the muscle-tendon unit as described in Chapter 2. In these indirect injuries often a preexisting chronic tendon injury has already weakened the tendon allowing the rupture to occur. In injury due to direct laceration the basic response is very similar to that described in acute ligament injuries. Inflammatory, proliferative, and maturation phases have clearly been identified in these injuries as well. Unlike ligaments, the healing of tendon injuries is often complicated by some of the unique features of tendon tissue. First, there is the constant tension on the tendon from the muscle that is attached to it. If the rupture or laceration is complete, the muscle tension will usually result in wide separation of the two torn tendon ends. Treatment needs to close the gap between these ends in order to allow satisfactory healing. In most tendon injuries this means a surgical repair of the tear or laceration. In addition, the tendon also needs to have a gliding function. Fibroblast proliferation from the surrounding tissue may be very effective in healing the defect in the injured tendon but at the same time causes scar tissue to develop between the tendon and the surrounding tissue. This scarring can eliminate the gliding motion of the tendon and thereby its function despite an otherwise healed tendon injury. The treatment of tendon injury therefore should be aimed at allowing and promoting the healing of the tendon tissue within itself but not to the surrounding tissues. Early mobilization of the healing tendon can accomplish this goal.

Acute Muscle Injuries

An acute muscle rupture, also called strain or pull, results in tearing of the muscle tissue as well as the connective tissue framework in and around the muscle fibers. Research has shown that a healthy muscle is most likely to tear very close to the muscle-tendon junction. The response to this injury is initially very similar to the response to acute ligament and tendon injuries. Initially there is bleeding, swelling, and disruption of muscle fiber and connective tissue. A pronounced inflammatory response develops within 24 to 48 hours (Fig. 3.4). Numerous inflammatory cells in the area of the rupture actively remove the injured and dead muscle fibers. The following phases differ somewhat from those of the healing response of tendon and ligament. Muscle fibers have the ability to regenerate. Young, emerging new muscle fibers or myotubes can be seen within several days in an attempt to replace the injured fibers that are being removed by the

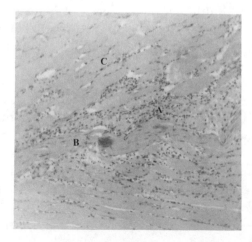

Figure 3.4 *Photomicrograph of infiltration of inflammatory cells (A) 48 hours after a partial tear of the junction between the tendon (B) and muscle (C).*

inflammatory cells (Fig. 3.5). At the same time fibroblasts from the surrounding connective tissue grow into the area similarly to tendon and ligament healing. In essence there is a competition between the regenerating muscle fibers and fibroblasts to fill the injured area. In adult patients the fibroblasts often gain more ground than the muscle fibers, which eventually results in a scar within the muscle tissue. As scar tissue has a different stiffness than muscle tissue, it is possible that such scar tissue is responsible for chronic pain or recurrences of strains which frequently occur in athletes.

A different type of muscle injury is a direct contusion. Often a blunt object, like the helmet of an opposing player, is responsible for this type of injury. This injury is often called a charley horse if it occurs in the quadriceps muscle. The injury response is initially very similar to that of a muscle strain. Acute hemorrhage and muscle fiber disruption are followed by inflammation and regeneration. Again, regeneration includes muscle fiber regeneration as well as a fibroblastic scar response. Occasionally, a further response is seen. Several weeks after the injury bone is formed in the injured area in severe contusions. This is called myositis ossificans (Fig. 3.6). It is not entirely clear why some cells in the injured area start producing this

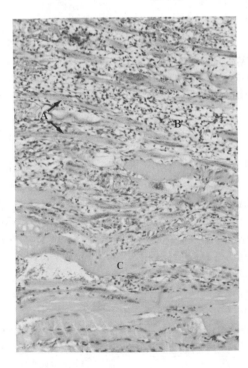

Figure 3.5 *Photomicrograph of regenerating myotubes (A) surrounded by inflammatory cells (B) and surviving muscle fibers (C) 5 days after a muscle tear.*

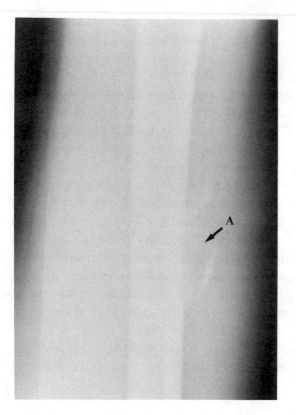

Figure 3.6 *X-ray of femur and thigh 2 months after a severe contusion showing the presence of myositis ossificans (A).*

bone. Some researchers have suggested that this means the underlying bone was injured at the time of the contusion, but this has not been proved conclusively. The bone formation will stop spontaneously but can cause significant pain and tightness in the affected muscle.

Acute Cartilage Injuries

Cartilage injuries should be divided into injuries to the joint or hyaline cartilage and those to meniscal or fibrocartilage.

Acute joint or hyaline cartilage injuries often occur as a result of "chipping off" a piece of cartilage in an otherwise healthy joint. Such a chondral lesion is occasionally accompanied by a chipped-off piece of bone, in which case it is called an osteochondral fracture (Fig. 3.7). The response to these cartilage injuries can be very different from that to ligament, tendon, and muscle injuries. The main reason for this difference appears to be the lack of blood supply in cartilage. If a chondral lesion does not affect the underlying bone, it appears that an injury response is virtually absent. There is no hemorrhage, no inflammatory cells appear, and the surrounding chondrocytes do not appear to be stimulated to heal the defect. This situation can even lead to further cartilage injury as the cartilage on the opposite side of the joint continuously rubs over this lesion. Secondary injury to the opposite cartilage as well as the edges of the original lesion can occur in this manner.

If the injury also involved the bone underlying the cartilage, as in an osteochondral fracture, the response can be quite different. The bone has good blood supply, and hemorrhage will occur into the lesion. This sets off a healing response. The chondrocytes in the surrounding cartilage are stimulated in this situation and migrate to the injured area. Usually they are capable of repairing the defect, although the new cartilage that will fill the defect is often of inferior quality. The repair tissue resembles fibrocartilage rather than hyaline cartilage.

Meniscal or fibrocartilage injuries are also dependent on the blood supply for their injury response. Most areas with fibrocartilage such as the meniscus in the knee joint have a limited blood supply. Some of the fibrocartilage lives on its own blood supply whereas other parts of the same meniscus have no blood supply (Fig. 3.8). Cartilage without blood supply receives its nutrients from the joint fluid by diffusion. Tears in the vascular portion result in hematoma formation and subsequent repair by surrounding chondrocytes with new fibrocartilage. This can result in complete healing of such an injury. Tears in the avascular region, again, do not seem to be able to evoke an adequate healing response. If left untreated, secondary injury to the surrounding tissues can also be possible as described previously.

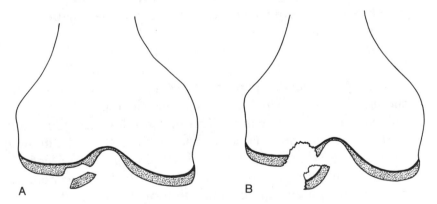

Figure 3.7 *Articular cartilage lesions. A cartilage injury can be confined to the cartilage only (A) or also involve the underlying bone (B).*

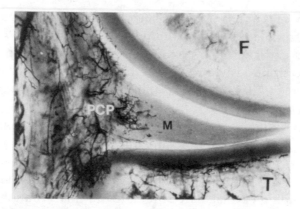

Figure 3.8 *Specially prepared histologic section showing the blood supply of the medial meniscus of the knee. The meniscus (M) is partially supplied by small blood vessels (PCP) and is located between femur (F) and tibia (T).* (Reproduced by permission from Arnoczky SP, Warren RF. Microvasculature of the human meniscus. Am J Sports Med 1982;10:90–95.)

Chronic Injuries

Significantly less is known about the response of soft tissue to chronic injuries. There is no good laboratory model for these injuries, and injuries in humans are generally treated nonsurgically, which makes it difficult to obtain more information on the healing response in these injuries.

Chronic ligament injuries are particularly poorly investigated. It is thought that repetitive stress can gradually attenuate some ligaments, as occasionally occurs in shoulder and elbow ligaments of throwing athletes. It is not known, however, whether this is actually accompanied by small tears in the ligament and actual inflammation as seen on a large scale in acute injuries.

Chronic tendon injuries are common. It appears that there are at least two distinct types of responses to chronic injury of the tendon. In one type, the tendon appears to be subjected to excessive, repetitive sliding or friction. This generally evokes a response from the outer lining or sheath of the tendon. This may result in actual inflammation in this area with production of fluid by the cells in the lining of this sheath. The athlete will notice this fluid buildup or edema. This condition is often called tendinitis or perhaps more appropriately paratenonitis, indicating inflammation of the sheath itself. With adequate rest and treatment the swelling and pain subside and allow normal use of the tendon again.

The other type of chronic tendon injury is a lesion within the tendon tissue itself. It seems to occur in tendons that are subjected to repetitive, high tensile stresses such as the Achilles tendon, patellar tendon, and rotator cuff. The most common location of this type of injury is near the attachment to the bone. There appears to be a breakdown of the internal tendon tissue in this location. The response to this injury seems different from that to an acute tendon injury. Surgical specimens from affected tendons do not appear to have any evidence of a significant inflammatory reaction. The histology mainly shows collagen fibril breakdown, ingrowth of some small blood vessels, but a very limited fibroblastic response (Fig. 3.9). Although this is often called tendinitis, it seems that this is not an appropriate name. The suffix "-itis" indicates inflammation, which appears to be lacking in these cases. The term tendinosis may be more appropriate. Many athletes with tendinosis will have chronic problems with pain owing to the very slow or even absent healing response. This is particularly a problem in the older athlete. This may indicate that aging of the tendon and repetitive stress are etiologic factors.

There is also relatively little known about chronic muscle injuries. It is not clear whether the previously described chronic compartment

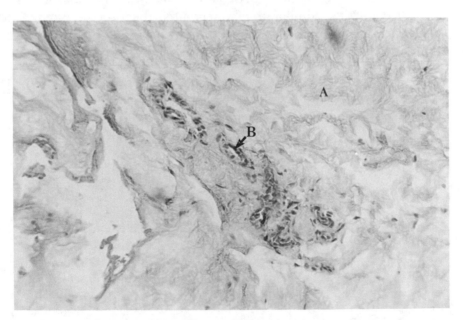

Figure 3.9 *Photomicrograph of tendon tissue excised at the time of surgery for chronic tendinosis. Disorganized collagen (A) and small blood vessel ingrowth (B) are seen without evidence of inflammatory cells.*

syndrome and delayed onset muscle soreness (see Chapter 2) truly represent chronic muscle injuries. They appear more subacute and temporary in nature. In delayed onset muscle soreness, repetitive eccentric contractions cause a diffuse inflammation on a microscopic level. Inflammatory cells are scattered throughout the muscle. There is also injury to the muscle fibers themselves. Isolated fibers lose their architecture and are later cleared away by inflammatory cells (Fig. 3.10). A fibroblastic response appears to be absent. Many investigators contend that the delayed onset muscle soreness is a way for the body to clear the muscle of aging, inferior muscle fibers. This is supported by the fact that on subsequent bouts of repeated eccentric exercise the delayed onset muscle soreness is lessened or even absent.

Finally, chronic injury can occur in any area where there is intense, repeated friction. This can be caused by movement of tendon over bone, tendon over other tendon, or skin over bone. Most of these areas develop a bursa. This is a thin-walled sac that contains a small amount of joint fluid–like material. The fluid is produced by the cells in the wall of the bursa. If the friction becomes excessive, a chronic injury can occur in and around the bursa. The cells in the wall produce excessive amounts of fluid, which results in pain and swelling in that area. Some mild inflammatory changes can also occur. This is called bursitis. Similar to paratenonitis, the process often resolves with a decrease in the friction and other anti-inflammatory treatment modalities.

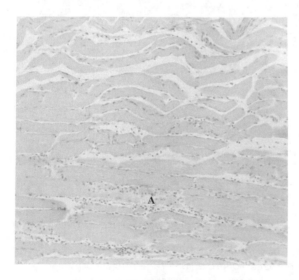

Figure 3.10 *Photomicrograph of delayed onset muscle soreness showing diffuse infiltration of inflammatory cells and only isolated muscle fiber necrosis (A).*

Suggested Readings

Arnoczky SP, Warren RF. Microvasculature of the human meniscus. Am J Sports Med 1982;10:90–95.

Finerman GAM, Noyes FR, eds. Biology and biomechanics of the traumatized synovial joint: the knee as a model. Rosemont, IL: American Academy of Orthopaedic Surgeons, 1992.

Frank C, Amiel D, Akeson WH. Healing of the medial collateral ligament of the knee: a morphological and biochemical assessment in rabbits. Acta Orthop Scand 1983;54:917–923.

Herring SA, Nilson KL. Introduction in overuse injuries. Clin Sports Med 1987;6(2):225–239.

Leadbetter WB, Buckwalter JA, Gordon SL. Sports induced inflammation. Park Ridge, IL: American Academy of Orthopaedic Surgeons, 1990.

Mankin HJ. The response of articular cartilage to mechanical injury. J Bone Joint Surg 1982;64A:460–466.

CHAPTER 4

Basic Principles of Treatment and Prevention of Soft Tissue Injuries

Louis C. Almekinders

Once the basic anatomy, biochemistry, mechanism of injury, and anticipated response to the soft tissue injury are known, a treatment plan can be formulated. Virtually all soft tissue injuries have a tendency to heal regardless of any attempt to intervene with a specific treatment. In some injuries this healing response can be extremely slow, and in others it can be quite rapid. The main objective of any treatment is to optimize the circumstances in which this healing takes place. This can be done by stimulating the beneficial parts of the injury response and by attempting to decrease the unfavorable parts of the response. For instance, inflammation may be needed in some cases to start the healing response but can be detrimental in other injuries because it causes pain and swelling.

At the same time one needs to define a good outcome for each injury in order to choose the optimal treatment methods. A ligament can be healed, but if it has healed in a stretched position, it will not be able to adequately perform its function. A good outcome in such a case is not only a healed but also a tight ligament. Certain treatment methods may stimulate part of the healing process but compromise the ultimate function and therefore may have to be avoided. Finally, one needs to consider prevention before releasing the athlete from treatment. Both recurrence of the original injury and injury to surrounding, previously uninjured structures are possible upon return to athletic activity. Both possibilities should be considered during treatment and rehabilitation.

Acute Ligament Injuries

Acute ligament ruptures or sprains generally cause immediate pain and swelling. As described in Chapter 3, inflammation will quickly develop in the ensuing days. The initial goal of the treatment is to control pain, swelling, and inflammation. Control of pain and swelling is advantageous because the athlete will be more comfortable and the inability to move the injured part will be minimized. Whether control of all the inflammation is absolutely needed is debatable. On the one hand, some of the inflammation is needed to clear away the injured cells and fibers so that healing can occur. On the other hand, it seems reasonable to assume that some of the abundant inflammation in acute injuries is excessive and even detrimental.

Accepted ways to control the excessive inflammation are physical modalities such as rest, ice compression, and elevation. These will be discussed in more detail in Chapter 5. In addition, medication is available that can affect the inflammatory response. Nonsteroidal anti-inflammatory drugs (NSAIDs) have been shown to suppress the inflammatory response in experimental situations. NSAIDs may do this by blocking the production of prostaglandins, one of the inflammatory mediators (Fig. 4.1). This inflammatory response is described in more detail in Chapter 3. It is also possible that NSAIDs are capable of affecting the inflammatory response by direct effects on the inflammatory cells. NSAIDs are also nonaddicting analgesics similar to acetaminophen.

In spite of their proposed anti-inflammatory effects, it remains uncertain how effective NSAIDs actually are in soft tissue inflammation due to injury. Some studies have failed to show any better results than other drugs such as acetaminophen. In addition, NSAIDs can

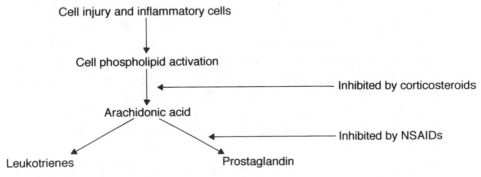

Figure 4.1 *One of the inflammatory pathways resulting in inflammatory mediators such as prostaglandins and leukotrienes.*

have significant side effects. Stomach erosion or ulceration as well as increased bleeding tendencies are some of the potential problems. In athletes with a history .of gastrointestinal ulcers, these drugs should not be used. If gastrointestinal problems develop during NSAID treatment, the drugs should be discontinued.

Currently, many NSAIDs are on the market (Table 4.1). Aspirin is, in fact, a type of NSAID. It is inexpensive and has been on the market for almost a century. To obtain not only analgesic but also anti-inflammatory effects from aspirin, it should be taken at a dose of at least 650 mg four times a day for an adult. Other over-the-counter NSAIDs available in the United States include ibuprofen and naproxen. Many other NSAIDs, available by prescription only, are being marketed. Their main advantage appears to be the twice-a-day or even once-a-day dosing. This may improve compliance in taking the medication as prescribed. Most studies fail to show a clear superiority of one NSAID over the others in soft tissue injuries. To obtain their maximal effects, it seems logical to start an NSAID as soon as possible after the injury and continue it for at least several days. Once the injury has moved into the proliferative and maturation phase, there seems to be little advantage to continuing the medication. Acetaminophen can be used at that point to control any residual pain.

Currently there are no other drugs that can be used routinely in the treatment of acute ligament injuries. Corticosteroid injections are not indicated in these injuries. Steroids are strong anti-inflammatory drugs but also seem to have significant side effects. Atrophy of otherwise healthy tissue can be seen with local steroid injection. Animal studies have shown mechanical weakening of tendon and ligaments especially with repeated steroid application. New research is focusing on the use of naturally occurring growth factors in ligament healing. Although some of the results are promising, it will be some time before these factors can be tried in actual ligament injuries.

As the inflammation subsides it becomes important to stimulate the proliferative response. Research has shown that motion stimulates this part of the injury response. Initiation of rehabilitative exercises and avoidance of prolonged immobilization are extremely important at that point. Often exercises can be started within several days after the injury. This is based on the premise that the affected joint is otherwise stable.

If the injury was severe enough to markedly destabilize the joint, another treatment approach may have to be followed before early motion can be initiated. Early motion in an unstable joint can lead to

Table 4.1   Most commonly used nonsteroidal anti-inflammatory drugs on the U.S. market

NAME (BRAND NAME)	RECOMMENDED DAILY DOSAGE
Salicylates	
Aspirin	325–650 mg, four times
Diflunisal (Dolobid)	500 mg, twice
Proprionic acids	
Ibuprofen (Nuprin, Advil, Brufen)	400–800 mg, four times
Naproxen (Naprosyn, Anaprox)	275–500 mg, twice
Flurbiprofen (Ansaid)*	100 mg, two or three times
Ketoprofen (Orudis)	50–75 mg, three or four times
Oxaprozin (Daypro)*	600–1200 mg, four times
Fenoprofen (Nalfon)	200 mg, four times
Indole/indene acetic acid	
Indomethacin (Indocin)	75 mg slow release, once
Sulindac (Clinoril)*	200 mg, twice
Etodolac (Lodine)	200–400 mg, three times
Aryl acetic acid	
Diclofenac (Voltaren)*	50–75 mg, two or three times
Heteraryl acetic acid	
Tolmetin (Tolectin)*	400 mg, three times
Oxicam	
Piroxicam (Feldene)*	20 mg, once
Fenamates	
Meclofenamate	50–100 mg, four times
Naphthylalkanone	
Nabumetone (Relafen)*	1000 mg, once

*Approved by the Food and Drug Administration for arthritis only.

a healed but lax and nonfunctional ligament. In these injuries the joint has to be restabilized first. This can be done by rigid immobilization in a cast or brace. However, this approach precludes the use of early motion. In most cases surgical repair or reconstruction of some or all of the injured ligaments can create a stable situation in which early motion is possible. This aggressive surgical intervention can result in excellent results without the ill effects of prolonged immobilization.

Once the injury moves from the proliferative phase to the maturation phase, further measures can be taken to improve the healing. Again, controlled motion can improve the rate and quality of healing. The athlete is guided from careful, protective rehabilitative exercises to more vigorous, sport-specific exercises. Chapter 5 will discuss this in more detail. Occasionally protection is still needed to prevent reinjury. Specially designed braces that allow continued exercise may be appropriate in this phase. Before return to full activities, the athlete's entire body should be rehabilitated. Many structures that were not originally part of the injury have often weakened from the relative inactivity during recovery. These structures, such as surrounding muscles and tendons, need to be rehabilitated in order to prevent injury to them upon return to sports. In addition, the athlete's psychomotor skills may have decreased making him or her prone to injury. To avoid these injuries, the rehabilitation should incorporate exercises that improve agility, technique, and judgment.

Acute Tendon Injuries

Acute disruption of tendons often requires aggressive surgical treatment to obtain a good functional result. After the injury the tension of the muscle attached to one side of the torn tendon will often cause a large separation between the two torn ends. Healing will be very difficult unless the torn ends are brought back together. Occasionally that is possible by positioning the limb in a particular manner. For instance, Achilles tendon ruptures can be approximated by placing the foot in a plantar-flexed position and the knee in a flexed position (Fig. 4.2). Unfortunately, this position must be maintained continuously for several weeks until enough healing has occurred that the ends will not separate anymore.

Prolonged immobilization, however, has many potential side effects. The muscles involved will atrophy and weaken significantly, and rehabilitation will take much longer. The healing tendon tissue will initially not be subjected to any stress if the injury is treated by immobilization. This stress can be helpful in aligning the new collagen in a parallel and more functional pattern. Finally, fibroblasts from the surrounding tissue will contribute to the healing response during full immobilization. This will cause scarring of the tendon to the surrounding tissue. Once healed, this can significantly impair the gliding

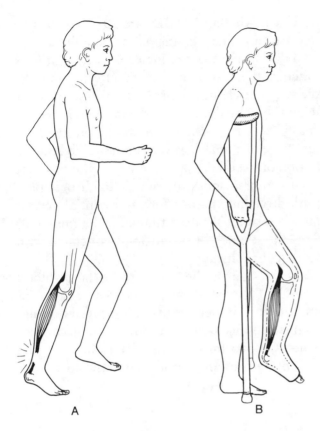

Figure 4.2 *An Achilles tendon rupture (A), subsequently treated by approximating the torn ends in a long leg cast (B).*

A

B

function of the involved tendon. For these reasons surgical repair of the torn or lacerated tendon ends is generally preferable. If a strong suture repair can be obtained at the time of surgery, there can be minimal immobilization, if any. Early motion can be initiated, which tends to result in a stronger, better-gliding tendon compared with the results of treatment by immobilization.

Acute Muscle Injuries

Both tears and contusions of the muscle are associated with a strong inflammatory response. As stated above, part of the inflammatory response is needed to clear away dead muscle fibers. However, some of the inflammatory response is probably excessive and makes early rehabilitation more difficult. Immediate initiation of rest, ice, compression, and elevation can help in this respect. Nonsteroidal anti-inflammatory drugs such as aspirin, ibuprofen, and naproxen are often used to amplify the anti-inflammatory treatment. As with ligament injuries, it is not clear whether NSAIDs are actually effective in this manner, but they are capable of giving adequate pain relief.

One of the main problems during the healing of muscle injuries is the tightening or contracture that can occur in the affected muscle. The athlete tends to keep the muscle in a shortened position in order to decrease the tension and thereby the pain in the muscle (Fig. 4.3). In addition, the fibroblastic scar response at the injury site tends to tighten with time. Contracture of a muscle is very undesirable because it limits the range of motion of the muscle and thereby of the adjacent joints. In addition, it seems to predispose the muscle to chronic pain and reinjury. Early, gentle stretching is therefore an essential part of the rehabilitation of muscle injuries. It also stimulates the muscle to heal faster and stronger without much of the atrophy associated with immobilization in a shortened position.

In partial muscle tears or strains, there is often a large blood collection within the muscle. Some studies suggest that removal of this hematoma with a needle and syringe results in improved healing. Some authors have also injected this area with drugs such as corticosteroids with good results. Corticosteroids can have significant side effects such as atrophy of the surrounding tissues. Until the advantage

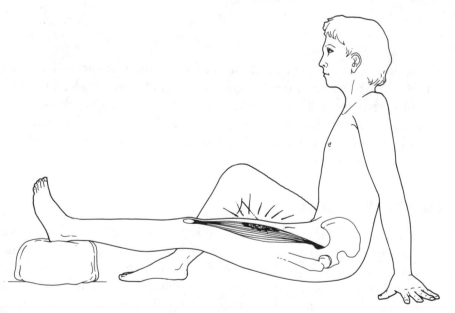

Figure 4.3 *Typical position of immobilization chosen by the athlete following a quadriceps muscle injury. Prolonged immobilization in this position leads to contracture and limited knee flexion.*

of steroid injection in this situation is clearly proved, it does not seem warranted to inject every muscle strain routinely.

In complete muscle tears the torn ends will widely separate owing to the constant tension within the muscle. Similar to tendon ruptures, early surgical repair is desirable in athletes. The repair will restore the proper anatomy and allow healing and often early rehabilitative exercises.

Acute Cartilage Injuries

As discussed in Chapter 3, cartilage injuries have a limited ability to heal. Unfortunately, there are only a few treatment forms to improve the healing potential. If a piece of cartilage is torn or chipped-off, it can mechanically interfere with the function of the joint. An otherwise smooth motion can become unpredictable as the loose piece moves around in the joint (Fig. 4.4). Surgical removal is often indicated to prevent further damage from this piece alone. Only in

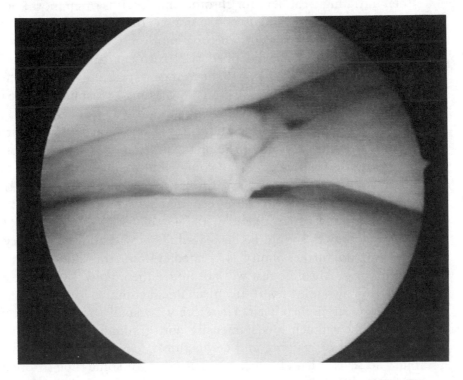

Figure 4.4 *Arthroscopic view of torn meniscal cartilage without evidence of healing.*

fibrocartilage with an adequate blood supply can these torn pieces sometimes be sutured back. An example of this is the peripheral meniscus tear of the knee.

There is invariably a remaining defect if the injured cartilage is removed. To improve the healing of this defect, two things can be attempted. If the defect does not extend into an area with blood supply, bleeding into the defect can be created surgically. Usually the bone underlying the defect is drilled, which causes bleeding into the defect. Research has shown that this can evoke a healing response with new fibrocartilage filling the defect. Unfortunately, this response can be unpredictable and incomplete. In addition to the drilling, the joint should be treated with early, nonstressful motion exercises. The motion has been shown to improve the fibrocartilage regeneration into the defect. Cartilage healing is quite slow, and many injuries can take 2 to 3 months to heal.

Chronic Injuries

When initiating treatment for chronic injuries, it is often most important to decide how and why the injury occurred. Many chronic injuries are from overuse or repetitive motion. Once the overuse and offending motion can be identified, the treatment can be initiated. The overuse can be very subtle. A slight change in training routine such as a switch from running on soft trails to running on asphalt can be the cause. A change in equipment such as shoes can also contribute to the injury. It is important to ask about any such changes that occurred not only around the time of the first symptoms but also well before that. Overuse injuries can take some time to build up. Once they cause symptoms they may have already been present for a long time but not severe enough to cause recognizable symptoms.

The mainstay of treatment in these athletes is relative rest. The offending activity should be decreased. This will allow the injury to heal, and no further injury is created. Often, this does not mean absolute rest. Absolute rest will not injure the involved structure any further but also takes away any mechanical stimulus for the structure to heal and strengthen itself. Therefore it is usually better to continue the sport at a much lower intensity and gradually build up to the original level of training and competition. Only occasionally is the injury so severe that absolute rest is needed for some time before any sport activity can be resumed.

During the period of relative rest and gradual buildup, the patient should be reminded of several things. Pain is the main guide in determining how much can be done. This means both pain during and pain after the workout. For instance, if the athlete still has pain running 1 mile, then he or she should start with workouts of $\frac{1}{2}$ to $\frac{3}{4}$ mile. Most workouts should be repeated two to three times before they are increased. Increases should be small such as 15% to 20% at one time. Only one thing should be increased at a time. Generally workout time is increased before intensity or speed is. Initially adequate rest should be given between workouts. Usually this is done by alternating rest days with workout days. Later during the rehabilitation this can be done by alternating easy and hard workout days. Finally, the athlete should be reminded that chronic injuries tend to heal much slower than acute injuries. Several months are sometimes needed before return to full activities. Even at that point, recurrences are still possible.

The program of relative rest and gradual return can be augmented with other forms of treatment. Nonsteroidal anti-inflammatory drugs can be of some help in treating the associated pain. It is unclear whether any of these injuries have a significant amount of inflammation despite names such as tendinitis, bursitis, and fasciitis. Therefore NSAIDs should not be relied on as the sole form of treatment in these chronic injuries. Rehabilitative exercises can be helpful in stimulating a chronically injured structure to heal. Stretching and strengthening should be an integral part of the rehabilitative program. Similarly, physical modalities such as ice, ultrasound, and massage can aid in the recovery from chronic injuries. These will be discussed in more detail in Chapter 5.

In some chronic injuries the use of corticosteroids appears to be beneficial. If the previously outlined program fails in cases of so-called tendinitis or fasciitis, it is reasonable to consider a local injection with a corticosteroid preparation (Table 4.2). It seems that this can break the vicious circle of irritation and pain and allow a more effective

Table 4.2   Commonly used corticosteroid prepartations on the U.S. market for parenteral use in soft tissue injuries

NAME (BRAND NAME)	RECOMMENDED DOSE
Triamcinolone acetonide (Aristocort)	5–40 mg
Triamcinolone hexacetonide (Aristospan)	2–20 mg
Betamethasone acetate (Celestone Soluspan)	2–6 mg
Methylprednisolone acetate (Depo-Medrol)	10–80 mg
Dexamethasone acetate (Decadron-LA)	4–16 mg

rehabilitation program. Several precautions should be considered when injecting corticosteroids. Because of the temporary weakening effects of the steroids, athletic activity should decreased or even avoided for at least 2 weeks following the injection. Activities can be gradually restarted after that period. Repeated injections should be avoided for the same reason. Reports of tendon ruptures associated with repeated steroid injections point to the potential risks. Most physicians will not inject steroids more than once every 3 to 4 months. The steroids should not be directly injected into the affected structure but rather around it. Injected directly into a tendon it may cause considerable weakening due to both the effects of the steroid itself and the increased pressure from the injected volume. Finally,

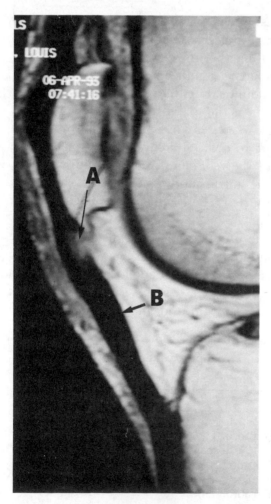

Figure 4.5 *Magnetic resonance imaging scan of a tendinosis lesion (A) in the patellar tendon (B), which may require surgical excision if not responsive to nonsurgical treatment.*

injection directly under the skin can cause permanent thinning and depigmentation of the skin and should be avoided.

In a limited number of chronic injuries, surgery may be needed to allow healing. Chronic tendon injuries, particularly forms of tendinosis (see Chapters 2 and 3), may not respond to any of the above-mentioned approaches. In those cases, surgery with excision of the degenerative areas in the tendon can lead to healing of the injury (Fig. 4.5). Chronic ligament injuries also may require surgical treatment. Chronic ligament injuries may be associated with gradual attenuation and laxity of the involved ligaments. This can lead to symptomatic instability of the involved joint. A surgical ligament-tightening procedure may be the only remaining choice to improve this condition.

Prevention of chronic injuries is an important part of the medical care of athletes. Rapid changes and increases in training regimens should be avoided. Appropriate, well-fitting protective equipment should be available when needed. Athletic shoes should have both adequate cushioning and support. Finally, all training and competition should be preceded by an adequate warm-up that includes flexibility exercises. Although the value of stretching has not been researched extensively, it seems to make good sense in the prevention of athletic injuries.

Suggested Readings

Almekinders LC. The efficacy of non-steroidal anti-inflammatory drugs in the treatment of ligament injuries. Sports Med 1990;9:137–142.

Almekinders LC. Anti-inflammatory treatment of muscular injuries in sports. Sports Med 1993;15:139–145.

Clancy WG. Specific rehabilitation for the injured recreational runner. Instr Course Lect 1989;28:483–486.

Cox YS. Current concepts in the role of steroids in the treatment of sprains and strains. Med Sci Sports Exerc 1984;16:216–217.

Kellet J. Acute soft tissue injuries; a review of the literature. Med Sci Sports Exerc 1986;18:489–500.

Woo LSY, Buckwalter JA, eds. Injury and repair of musculoskeletal tissues. Park Ridge, IL: American Academy of Orthopaedic Surgeons, 1988.

CHAPTER 5

Principles of Rehabilitation

William E. Prentice

One of the primary goals of every sports medicine professional is to create a playing environment for the athlete that is as safe as it can possibly be. Regardless of that effort, the nature of athletic participation dictates that injuries will eventually occur. Fortunately, few of the injuries that occur in an athletic setting are life-threatening. The majority are not serious and lend themselves to rapid rehabilitation. When injuries do occur the focus of the sports therapist shifts from injury prevention to injury treatment and rehabilitation.

The process of rehabilitation begins immediately following injury. Initial first aid and management techniques can have a substantial effect on the course and ultimate outcome of the rehabilitative process. Thus, in addition to possessing sound understanding of how injuries can be prevented, the sports therapist must be competent in providing correct and appropriate initial care when injury does occur.

Designing programs for rehabilitation is relatively simple and involves several basic short-term goals: (1) controlling initial swelling and pain, (2) maintaining or improving flexibility, (3) returning or increasing strength, (4) reestablishing neuromuscular control, and (5) maintaining levels of cardiorespiratory fitness. The long-term goal is

Sections from this chapter were reprinted by permission from Prentice WE, ed. Rehabilitation techniques in sports medicine. St. Louis: CV Mosby, 1994. Lephart S. Reestablishing proprioception, kinesthesia, joint position sense, and neuromuscular control in rehabilitation (pages 118 to 135). McGee M. Functional progressions in rehabilitation (pages 181 to 194). Selepak G. Aquatic therapy in rehabilitation (pages 195 to 203).

to return the injured athlete to practice or competition as quickly and safely as possible. This is the easy part of supervising a rehabilitation program. The difficult part is knowing exactly when and how to change or alter the rehabilitation protocols to most effectively accomplish both long-term and short-term goals.

The approach to rehabilitation in a sports medicine environment differs considerably from that in most other rehabilitation settings. The competitive nature of athletics necessitates an aggressive approach to rehabilitation. As the competitive season in most sports is relatively short, the athlete does not have the luxury of being able to simply wait until the injury heals. The goal is to return to activity as soon and as safely as possible. Thus the sports therapist who is supervising the rehabilitation program must walk a thin line between not pushing the athlete hard enough or fast enough, and being overly aggressive. In either case, a mistake in judgment on the part of the sports therapist may hinder the athlete's return to activity.

Decisions of when and how to alter and progress a rehabilitation program should be based within the framework of the healing process. The sports therapist must possess a sound understanding of both the sequence and time frames for the various phases of healing, realizing that certain physiologic events must occur during each of the phases. Anything done during a rehabilitation program that interferes with this healing process will most likely increase the time required for rehabilitation and slow the return to full activity. The healing process must have an opportunity to accomplish what it is supposed to. At best the sports therapist can only try to create an environment that is conducive to the healing process. Little can be done to speed up that process physiologically, but there are many things that may be done during rehabilitation that impede healing.

Sports therapists have many tools that can facilitate the rehabilitative process. How they choose to utilize these tools is often a matter of individual preference and experience. Furthermore, each patient is a little different, and the patient's response to various treatment protocols is somewhat variable. Thus it is impossible to determine specific protocols that can be followed like a recipe. In fact, use of rehabilitation "recipes" should be strongly discouraged. Rather, the sports therapist must develop a broad theoretical knowledge base from which specific techniques of rehabilitation may be selected and practically applied to each individual patient.

Managing the Healing Process Through Rehabilitation

In sports medicine, the rehabilitation philosophy relative to inflammation and healing following injury is to assist the natural processes of the body while doing no harm. The course of rehabilitation chosen by the sports therapist must utilize knowledge of the healing process and its therapeutic modifiers to guide, direct, and stimulate the structural function and integrity of the injured part. The primary goal should be to have a positive influence on the process of inflammation and repair to expedite recovery of function in terms of range of motion, muscular strength and endurance, neuromuscular control, and cardiorespiratory endurance. The sports therapist must try to minimize the early effects of excessive inflammatory processes including pain modulation, edema control, and reduction of associated muscle spasm, which can produce loss of joint motion and contracture. Finally, the sports therapist should concentrate on preventing the recurrence of injury by influencing the structural ability of the injured tissue to resist future overloads by incorporating various training techniques. The subsequent sections in this chapter can serve as a guide in utilizing the many different rehabilitation tools available.

Initial Management of Acute Injuries

Initial first aid and management techniques are perhaps the most critical part of any rehabilitation program. The initial management unquestionably has a significant effect on the course of the rehabilitative process. Regardless of the type of injury, the one problem they all have in common is swelling. Swelling may be caused by any number of factors including bleeding, production of synovial fluid, an accumulation of inflammatory by-products, and edema (which is nothing more than an accumulation of body fluid), or by a combination of several factors. No matter which mechanism is involved, swelling produces an increased pressure in the injured area, and increased pressure causes pain. Swelling can also cause neuromuscular inhibition, which results in weak muscle contraction. Swelling is most likely during the first 72 hours after an injury. Once swelling has occurred, the healing process is significantly retarded. The injured area cannot return to normal until all the swelling is gone.

Therefore everything that is done in terms of first aid management of any of these conditions should be directed toward controlling the

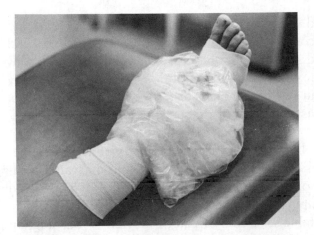

Figure 5.1 *Musculoskeletal injuries should be treated initially with restricted activity, ice, compression, and elevation.*

swelling. If the swelling can be controlled initially in the acute stage of injury, the time required for rehabilitation is likely to be significantly reduced. To control and severely limit the amount of swelling, the RICE principle—restricted activity, ice, compression, and elevation—can be applied (Fig. 5.1). Each factor plays a critical role in limiting swelling, and all should be used simultaneously.

Restricted Activity

Rest following any type of injury is an extremely important component of any treatment program. Once an anatomic structure is injured, it immediately begins the process of healing. If the injured structure is not rested and is subjected to external stress and strains, there is no opportunity for the healing process to occur. Consequently, the injury does not get better, and the time required for rehabilitation is markedly increased. The number of days necessary for resting varies with the severity of the injury, but patients with most minor injuries should rest them for approximately 48 to 72 hours before an active rehabilitation program is begun.

It must be emphasized that rest does not mean that the athlete does nothing. The term "rest" applies only to the injured body part. During this period, the athlete should continue to work on cardiovascular fitness and on strengthening and flexibility exercises for the other parts of the body not affected by the injury.

Ice

The use of cold is the initial treatment of choice for virtually all conditions involving injuries to the musculoskeletal system. It is most commonly used immediately after injury to decrease pain and promote local vasoconstriction, thus controlling hemorrhage and edema. It is also used in the acute phase of inflammatory conditions such as bursitis, tenosynovitis, and tendinitis, in which heat may cause further pain and swelling. Cold is also used to reduce the reflex muscle spasm and spastic conditions that accompany pain. Its analgesic effect is probably one of its greatest benefits. One explanation of the analgesic effect is that cold decreases the velocity of nerve conduction, although it does not entirely eliminate it. Cold may also bombard cutaneous sensory nerve receptor areas with so many cold impulses that pain impulses are lost. With ice treatments, the athlete reports an uncomfortable sensation of cold, followed by burning, an aching sensation, and finally complete numbness.

Because of the low thermal conductivity of underlying subcutaneous fat tissues, applications of cold for short periods are ineffective in cooling deeper tissues. For this reason longer treatments of 20 to 30 minutes are recommended. Cold treatments are generally believed to be more effective in reaching deeper tissues than most forms of heat. Cold applied to the skin is capable of significantly lowering the temperature of tissues at a considerable depth. The extent of this lowered tissue temperature depends on the type of cold applied to the skin, the duration of its application, the thickness of the subcutaneous fat, and the region of the body to which it is applied. Ice should be applied to the injured area until the signs and symptoms of inflammation have disappeared and there is little or no chance that swelling will be increased by using some form of heat. Ice should be used for at least 72 hours after an acute injury.

Compression

Compression is probably the single most important technique for controlling initial swelling. The purpose of compression is to mechanically reduce the amount of space available for swelling by applying pressure around an injured area. The best way of applying pressure is to use an elastic wrap (such as an Ace bandage) to apply firm but even pressure around the injury.

Because of the pressure buildup in the tissues, having a compression wrap in place for a long time may become painful. Despite significant pain, however, the wrap must be kept in place because it is so important in the control of swelling. The compression wrap should be left in place continuously for at least 72 hours after an acute injury.

In many overuse problems that involve ongoing inflammation, such as tendinitis, tenosynovitis, and particularly bursitis, the compression wrap should be worn until the swelling is almost entirely gone.

Elevation

The fourth factor that assists in controlling swelling is elevation. The injured part, particularly an extremity, should be elevated to eliminate the effects of gravity on blood pooling in the extremities. Elevation assists venous drainage of blood and other fluids from the injured area back to the central circulatory system. The greater the degree of elevation, the more effective the reduction in swelling. For example, in an ankle sprain, the leg should be placed in such a position that the ankle is virtually straight up in the air. The injured part should be elevated as much as possible during the first 72 hours.

The appropriate technique for initial management of the acute injuries discussed in this chapter, regardless of where they occur, would be the following:

1. Apply a compression wrap directly over the injury. Wrapping should be from distal to proximal. Tension should be firm and consistent. Wetting the elastic wrap to facilitate the passage of cold from ice packs may be helpful.

2. Surround the injured area entirely with ice bags and secure them in place. Ice bags should be left on for 45 minutes initially and then 1 hour off and 30 minutes on as much as possible over the next 24 hours. During the following 48-hour period, ice should be applied as often as possible.

3. The injured part should be elevated as much as possible during the initial 72-hour period after injury. Keeping the injury elevated while sleeping is particularly important.

4. Allow the injured part to rest for approximately 72 hours following the injury.

Techniques of Reconditioning and Therapeutic Exercise

The sports therapist is responsible for designing, monitoring, and progressing programs of rehabilitation for injured athletes. The goals for patients in a sports medicine rehabilitation program differ from the goals for other patient populations. The athlete must return to competitive fitness levels, and the intensity of the rehabilitation must be adjusted appropriately during the course of the program. The sports therapist has to understand the principles and techniques involved in reconditioning the injured athlete. The term therapeutic exercise is commonly used to refer to techniques of reconditioning.

Flexibility

Flexibility has been defined as the ability to move a joint or series of joints through a full, nonrestricted, pain-free range of motion. For the sports therapist, a return to or improvement on this preinjury range is an important goal of any rehabilitation program. Most sports therapists would agree that good flexibility is essential to successful physical performance although their ideas are based primarily on observation rather than scientific research. They also believe that maintaining good flexibility is important in prevention of injury to the musculotendinous unit, and they will generally insist that stretching exercises be included as part of the warm-up before the patient engages in strenuous activity although little or no research evidence is available to support this practice (Fig. 5.2).

Flexibility is specific to a given joint or movement. A person may have good range of motion in the ankles, knees, hips, back, and one shoulder joint. If the other shoulder joint lacks normal movement, however, then a problem exists that needs to be corrected before the person can function normally. Flexibility may be limited by a number of factors including normal anatomic bony structure, fat, skin, muscles and their tendons, and connective tissue.

Active and Passive Range of Motion

Active range of motion, also called dynamic flexibility, refers to the degree to which a joint can be moved by a voluntary contraction of the muscles surrounding that joint. Dynamic flexibility is not necessarily a good indicator of the stiffness or looseness of a joint because it depends not only on joint flexibility but also on muscle strength and control.

Passive range of motion, sometimes called static flexibility, refers to the degree to which a joint may be passively moved to the endpoints in the range of motion. No muscle contraction is involved to move a joint through a passive range.

When a muscle actively contracts, it produces a joint movement through a specific range of motion. However, if passive pressure is

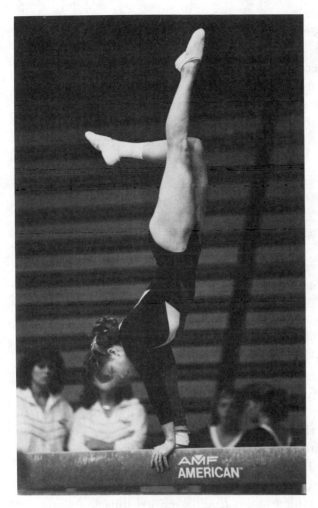

Figure 5.2 *Flexibily is a key component for successful performance and in reducing the likelihood of injury in many athletic activities.*

applied to an extremity, it is capable of moving farther in the range of motion. It is essential in sport activities that an extremity be capable of moving through a nonrestricted range of motion. For example, a hurdler who cannot fully extend the knee joint in a normal stride is at considerable disadvantage because stride length and thus speed will be reduced significantly.

Stretching Techniques

The goal of any effective flexibility program should be to improve the range of motion at a given joint by altering the extensibility of the musculotendinous units that produce movement at that joint. It is well documented that exercises that stretch these musculotendinous units over a period of time will increase the range of movement possible around a given joint.

Stretching techniques for improving flexibility have evolved over the years. The oldest technique for stretching is called ballistic stretching, which makes use of repetitive bouncing motions. A second technique, known as static stretching, involves stretching a muscle to the point of discomfort and then holding it at the point for an extended time. This technique has been used for many years. Recently another group of stretching techniques known collectively as proprioceptive neuromuscular facilitation (PNF), involving alternating contractions and stretches, has also been recommended. Researchers have had considerable discussion about which of these techniques is most effective for improving range of motion.

Ballistic Stretching

If one were to walk out to the track on any spring or fall afternoon and watch people who are warming up to run, they would probably be using bouncing movements to stretch particular muscles. This bouncing technique is more appropriately known as ballistic stretching, in which repetitive contractions of the agonist muscle are used to produce quick stretches of the antagonist muscle.

Over the years, many fitness experts have questioned the safety of the ballistic stretching technique. Their concerns have been based primarily on the idea that ballistic stretching creates somewhat uncontrolled forces within the muscle that may exceed the extensibility limits of the muscle fiber, thus producing small microtears within the musculotendinous unit. Certainly this may be true in sedentary persons or perhaps in athletes who have sustained muscle injuries.

Most sport activities are dynamic and require ballistic-type movements. For example, forcefully kicking a soccer ball 50 times involves a repeated dynamic contraction of the agonist quadriceps muscle. The antagonist hamstrings are contracting eccentrically to decelerate the lower leg. Ballistic stretching of the hamstring muscles before engaging in this type of activity should allow the muscle to gradually adapt to the imposed demands and reduce the likelihood of injury. Because ballistic stretching is more functionally related to the sports activity, it should be integrated into both training and reconditioning programs when appropriate.

Static Stretching

Static stretching is another extremely effective and popular stretching technique. This technique involves passively stretching a given antagonist muscle by placing it in a position of maximal stretch and holding it there for an extended time. Recommendations for the optimal time for holding this stretched position vary, ranging from as short as 3 seconds to as long as 60 seconds. Stretches lasting for longer than 30 seconds seem to be uncomfortable for the athlete. A static stretch of each muscle should be repeated three or four times. A static stretch may be accomplished by using a contraction of the agonist muscle to place the antagonist in a position of stretch. A passive static stretch requires the use of body weight or assistance from the sports therapist or a partner.

Much research has been done comparing ballistic and static stretching techniques for the improvement of flexibility. It has been shown that static and ballistic stretching appear to be about equally effective in increasing flexibility and that there is no significant difference between the two. However, much of the literature states that with static stretching there is less danger of exceeding the extensibility limits of the involved joints because the stretch is more controlled. Most of the literature seems to indicate that ballistic stretching is apt to cause muscular soreness, especially in sedentary persons, whereas static stretching generally does not and therefore is commonly used in injury rehabilitation of sore or strained muscles.

Static stretching is most likely a much safer stretching technique, especially for sedentary or untrained individuals. However, as many physical activities involve dynamic movement, warm-up stretching should begin with static stretching and continue with ballistic stretching, which more closely resembles the dynamic activity.

Proprioceptive Neuromuscular Facilitation

PNF stretching techniques were first used by physical therapists for treating patients who had various types of neuromuscular disorders. Only recently have PNF exercises been used as a stretching technique for increasing flexibility.

Several different PNF techniques are currently being used for stretching, including slow-reversal-hold-relax, contract-relax, and hold-relax techniques. All involve some combination of alternating isometric or isotonic contractions and relaxation of both agonist and antagonist muscles (a 10-second pushing phase followed by a 10-second relaxing phase). PNF stretching techniques can be used to stretch any muscle in the body. They are perhaps best performed with a partner although they may also be done using a wall as resistance (Fig. 5.3).

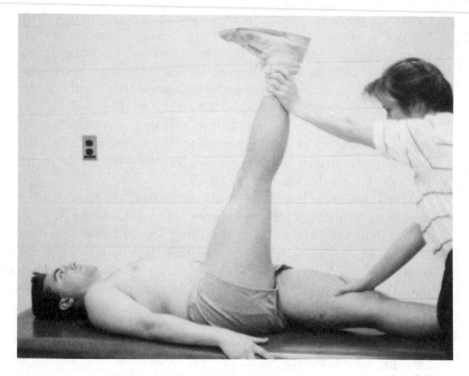

Figure 5.3 *Proprioceptive neuromuscular facilitation stretching techniques are an effective means of increasing range of motion.*

Muscular Strength, Endurance, and Power

One of the primary rehabilitation program goals of any sports therapist is to return the athlete to preinjury levels of muscular strength and endurance. The development of muscular strength is an essential component of any reconditioning program. By definition, strength is the ability of a muscle to generate force against some resistance. Maintenance of at least a normal level of strength in a given muscle or muscle group is important for normal healthy living. Muscle weakness or imbalance can result in abnormal movement or gait and can impair normal functional movement. Muscle weakness can also produce poor posture.

Muscular strength is closely associated with muscular endurance. Muscular endurance is the ability to perform repetitive muscular contractions against some resistance for an extended period of time. As muscular strength increases, there tends to be a corresponding increase in endurance. For example, a person can lift a weight 25 times. If muscular strength is increased by 10% through weight training, it is very likely that the maximal number of repetitions would be increased because it is easier for the person to lift the weight. For most people, developing muscular endurance is more important than developing muscular strength because muscular endurance is probably more critical in carrying out the everyday activities of living. This becomes increasingly true with age. However, a tremendous amount of strength is necessary for anyone involved in some type of sports competition.

Most movements in sports are explosive and must include elements of both strength and speed if they are to be effective. If a large amount of force is generated quickly, the movement can be referred to as a power movement. Without the ability to generate power, an athlete will be limited in his or her performance capabilities.

Strength training plays a critical role both in achieving competitive fitness levels and in injury rehabilitation.

Types of Skeletal Muscle Contraction

Skeletal muscle is capable of three different types of contraction: (1) an isometric contraction, (2) a concentric contraction, and (3) an eccentric contraction. An isometric contraction occurs when the muscle contracts to produce tension, but there is no change in length of the muscle. Considerable force can be generated against some immovable resistance even though no movement occurs. In a concentric contraction the muscle shortens in length as tension is developed to overcome or move some resistance. In an eccentric contraction, the resistance is greater than the muscular force being produced and the muscle lengthens while producing tension. Concentric and eccentric contractions are both considered to be dynamic movements.

Techniques of Resistance Training

Techniques of resistance training for strength improvement include isometric exercise, progressive resistive exercise, isokinetic training, circuit training, and plyometric excercise. Regardless of which of these techniques is used, one basic principle of reconditioning is extremely important. For a muscle to improve in strength, it must be forced to work at a higher level than that to which it is accustomed. In other words, it must be overloaded. Without overload the muscle will be able to maintain strength as long as training is continued against a resistance to which the muscle is accustomed. However, no further strength gains will be realized. This maintenance of existing levels of muscular strength may be more important in weight-training programs that emphasize muscular endurance rather than strength gains. It is certainly true that many can benefit more in terms of overall health by concentrating on improving muscular endurance. However, to most effectively build muscular strength, weight training requires a consistent, increasing effort against progressively increasing resistance.

Resistive exercise is based primarily on the principles of overload and progression. If these principles are applied, all of the following training techniques will improve muscular strength over a period of time.

In a rehabilitation setting, progressive overload is limited to some degree by the healing process. Because the sports therapist takes an aggressive approach to rehabilitation, the rate of progression is perhaps best determined by the injured athlete's response to a specific exercise. Exacerbation of pain or increased swelling should signal the sports therapist that the rate of progression is too aggressive.

Isometric Exercise

An isometric exercise involves a muscle contraction in which the length of the muscle remains constant while tension develops toward a maximal force against an immovable resistance. Isometric exercises are capable of increasing muscular strength. However, strength gains are relatively specific, with only about 20° overflow to the joint angle at which training is performed. At other angles, the strength curve drops off dramatically because of a lack of motor activity at that angle. Thus strength is increased at the specific angle of exertion, but there is no corresponding increase in strength at other positions in the range of motion.

Another major disadvantage of these isometric exercises is that they tend to produce a spike in systolic blood pressure that can result in potentially life-threatening cardiovascular accidents. This sharp increase in systolic blood pressure results from a Valsalva maneuver, which increases intrathoracic pressure. To avoid or minimize this effect, it is recommended that normal breathing is not interrupted during the maximal contraction to prevent this increase in pressure.

Isometric exercises are widely used in injury rehabilitation or reconditioning. A number of conditions or ailments resulting from either trauma or overuse must be treated with strengthening exercises.

Unfortunately, these problems may be exacerbated with full-range-of-motion strengthening exercises. It may be more desirable to make use of positional isometric exercises until the healing process has progressed to the point that full-range activities can be performed. During rehabilitation, it is often recommended that a muscle be contracted isometrically for 10 seconds at a time, at a frequency of 10 or more contractions per hour.

Progressive Resistive Exercise

A second technique of resistance training is perhaps the most commonly used and most popular technique among sports therapists for improving muscular strength in a reconditioning program. Progressive resistive exercise training uses exercises that strengthen muscles through a contraction that overcomes some fixed resistance such as with dumbbells, barbells, or various weight machines. Progressive resistive exercise uses isotonic contractions in which force is generated while the muscle is changing in length.

Isotonic contractions may be either concentric or eccentric. In performing a biceps curl, for one to lift the weight from the starting position, the biceps muscle must contract and shorten in length. This shortening contraction is referred to as a concentric or positive contraction. If the biceps muscle does not remain contracted when the weight is being lowered, gravity will cause this weight to simply fall back to the starting position. Thus to control the weight as it is being lowered, the biceps muscle must continue to contract while at the same time gradually lengthening. A contraction in which the muscle is lengthening while still applying force is called an eccentric or negative contraction. It is possible to generate greater amounts of force against resistance with an eccentric contraction than with a concentric contraction.

Traditionally, progressive resistive exercise has concentrated primarily on the concentric component without paying much attention to the importance of the eccentric component. The use of eccentric contractions, particularly in rehabilitation of various injuries related to sports, has received considerable emphasis in recent years. Eccentric contractions are critical for deceleration of limb motion especially during high-velocity dynamic activities. For example, a baseball pitcher relies on an eccentric contraction of the external rotators of the glenohumeral joint to decelerate the humerus, which may be internally rotating at speeds as high as 8000° per second. Certainly, strength deficits or the inability of a muscle to tolerate these eccentric forces can predispose it to injury. Thus in a rehabilitation program the sports therapist should incorporate eccentric strengthening exercises. Eccentric contractions are possible with all free weights, with the majority of isotonic exercise machines, and with most isokinetic devices. Eccentric contractions are used with plyometric exercise and may also be incorporated with functional PNF strengthening patterns.

Isotonic Exercise Equipment

Various types of exercise equipment can be used with progressive resistive exercise including free weights (barbells and dumbbells) or exercise machines such as Universal, Nautilus, Eagle, Body Master, Keiser, Paramount, Continental, Pyramid, Sprint, Hydrafitness, Dynatrac, Future, and Bull, to list a few. Dumbbells and barbells require the use of iron plates of varying weights that can be easily changed by adding or subtracting equal amounts of weight to both sides of the bar. The exercise machines for the most part have a stack of weights that are lifted through a series of levers or pulleys. The stack of weights slides up and down on a pair of bars that restrict the movement to only one plane. Weight can be increased or decreased simply by changing the position of a weight key (Fig. 5.4).

There are advantages and disadvantages to both the free weights and machines. The machines are relatively safe to use in comparison with free weights. For example, a bench press with free weights requires that a partner help lift the weight back onto the support racks if there is not enough strength to complete the lift; otherwise, the weight may be dropped on the chest. With the machines the weight may be easily and safely dropped without fear of injury. It is also a simple process to increase or decrease the weight by moving a single weight key with the exercise machines, although changes can generally be made only in increments of 10 or 15 pounds. With free weights, iron plates must be added or removed from each side of the barbell.

Surgical tubing as a means of providing resistance has been widely used in sports medicine. The advantage of exercising with surgical tubing is that the direction of movement is less restricted than with either free weights or the exercise machines. Thus exercise can be done against resistance in more functional movement planes.

Regardless of which type of equipment is used, the same principles of progressive resistive exercise may be applied. In progressive resis-

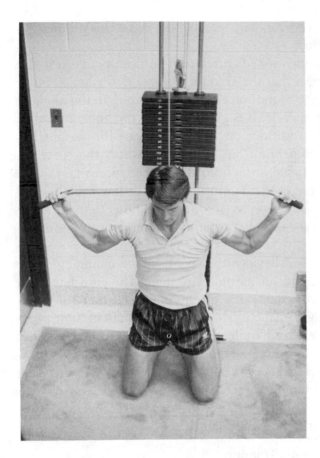

Figure 5.4 *Strength training is an essential component of all injury rehabilitation programs.*

tive exercise it is essential to incorporate both concentric and eccentric contractions. Research has clearly demonstrated that the muscle should be overloaded and fatigued both concentrically and eccentrically for the greatest strength improvement to occur.

When training specifically for the development of muscular strength, the concentric portion of the exercise should require 1 to 2 seconds while the eccentric portion of the lift should require 2 to 4 seconds. The ratio of the concentric component to the eccentric component should be approximately 1:2. Physiologically the muscle will fatigue much more rapidly concentrically than eccentrically. Athletes who have strength-trained using both free weights and the exercise machines realize the difference in the amount of weight that can be lifted. Unlike the machines, free weights have no restricted motion and can thus move in many different directions, depending on the forces applied. With free weights, an element of muscular control on the part of the lifter to prevent the weight from moving in any direction other than vertical will usually decrease the amount of weight that can be lifted.

One problem often mentioned in relation to progressive resistive exercise reconditioning is that the amount of force necessary to move a weight through a range of motion changes according to the angle of pull of the contracting muscle. It is greatest when the angle of pull is approximately 90°. In addition, once the inertia of the weight has been overcome and momentum has been established, the force required to move the resistance varies according to the force that muscle can produce through the range of motion. Thus it has been argued that a disadvantage of any type of isotonic exercise is that the force required to move the resistance is constantly changing throughout the range of movement.

Nautilus attempted to alleviate this problem of changing force capabilities by using a cam in its pulley system. The cam has been individually designed for each piece of equipment so that the resistance is variable throughout the movement. It attempts to alter resistance so that the muscle can handle a greater load, but at the points where the joint angle or muscle length is mechanically disadvantageous, it reduces the resistance to muscle movement. Whether this design does what the manufacturer claims is debatable. This change in resistance at different points in the range has been labeled accommodating resistance, or variable resistance.

Specific Techniques of Strength Training

Perhaps the single most confusing aspect of progressive resistive exercise is the terminology used to describe specific programs. The following list of terms with their operational definitions may help clarify the confusion:

- ✗ *Repetitions*: number of times one repeats a specific movement
- ✗ *Repetition maximum*: maximum number of repetitions at a given weight
- ✗ *Set*: a particular number of repetitions
- ✗ *Intensity*: the amount of weight or resistance lifted
- ✗ *Recovery period*: the rest interval between sets
- ✗ *Frequency*: the number of times an exercise is done in a week

Specific recommendations for techniques of improving muscular strength are controversial among sports therapists. A considerable amount of research has been done in the area of resistance training relative to (1) the amount of weight to be used, (2) the number of repetitions, (3) the number of sets, and (4) the frequency of training.

A variety of specific programs have been proposed that recommend the optimal amount of weight, number of sets, number of repetitions, and frequency for producing maximal gains in levels of muscular strength. Specific programs include the DeLorme technique, the Oxford technique, MacQueen's technique, the Sander's program, Knight's DAPRE program, and Berger's program.

Regardless of the techniques used, however, the healing process must dictate the specifics of any strength-training program. Certainly to improve strength the muscle must be overloaded. The amount of weight used and the number of repetitions must be enough to make the muscle work at higher intensity than it is used to working. This factor is the most critical in any strength-training program. The strength-training program must also be designed to ultimately meet the specific competitive needs of the athlete.

For rehabilitation purposes, strengthening exercises should be performed on a daily basis initially, with the amount of weight, number of sets, and number of repetitions governed by the injured athlete's response to the exercise. As the healing process progresses and pain or swelling is no longer an issue, a particular muscle or muscle group should be exercised consistently every other day. At that point, the frequency of weight training should be at least three times per week but no more than four times per week. It must also be added that it is common for serious weight lifters to lift every day; however, they exercise different muscle groups on successive days. For example, Monday, Wednesday, and Friday may be used for upper body muscles, whereas Tuesday, Thursday, and Saturday are used for lower body muscles.

Isokinetic Exercise

An isokinetic exercise involves a muscle contraction in which the length of the muscle is changing while the contraction is performed at a constant velocity. In theory, maximal resistance is provided throughout the range of motion by the machine. The resistance provided by the machine will move only at some preset speed regardless of the torque applied to it by the individual. Thus the key to isokinetic exercise is not the resistance, but the speed at which resistance can be moved.

Several isokinetic devices are available commercially; the Ariel Computerized Exercise System, Cybex, Orthotron, Biodex, KinCom,

Lido, MERAC, and Mini-gym are among the more common isokinetic devices. In general, they rely on hydraulic, pneumatic, and mechanical pressure systems to produce this constant velocity of motion. The majority of the isokinetic devices are capable of resisting both concentric and eccentric contractions at a fixed speed to exercise a muscle.

Isokinetics as a Conditioning Tool

Isokinetic devices are designed so that regardless of the amount of force applied against a resistance, it can only be moved at a certain speed. That speed will be the same whether maximal force or only half the maximal force is applied. Consequently, when training isokinetically, it is absolutely necessary to exert as much force against the resistance as possible (maximal effort) for maximal strength gains to occur. This is one of the major problems with an isokinetic strength-training program.

Anyone who has been involved in a weight-training program knows that on some days it is difficult to find the motivation to work out. Because isokinetic training requires a maximal effort, it is very easy to "cheat" and not go through the workout at a high level of intensity. In a progressive resistive exercise program, the athlete knows how much weight has to be lifted with how many repetitions. Thus isokinetic training is often more effective if a partner system is used, primarily as a means of motivation toward maximal effort.

When isokinetic training is done properly with maximal effort, it is theoretically possible that maximal strength gains are best achieved through the isokinetic training method in which the velocity and force of the resistance are the same throughout the range of motion. However, there is no conclusive research to support this theory.

Whether this changing force capability is in fact a deterrent to improving the ability to generate force against some resistance is debatable. It must be remembered that in real life it does not matter whether the resistance is changing; what is important is that an individual develops enough strength to move objects from one place to another. The amount of strength necessary for athletes is largely dependent on their level of competition.

Another major disadvantage of using isokinetic devices as a conditioning tool is their cost. With initial purchase costs ranging between $40,000 and 60,000, and the necessity of regular maintenance and software upgrades, the use of an isokinetic device for general conditioning or resistance training is, for the most part, unrealistic. Thus isokinetics is primarily used as a diagnostic and rehabilitative tool.

Isokinetics in Rehabilitation

Isokinetic strength testing gained a great deal of popularity throughout the 1980s in rehabilitation settings. This is primarily because it provides an objective means of quantifying existing levels of muscular strength and thus is useful as a diagnostic tool.

Because the capability exists for training at specific speeds, the relative advantages of training at fast or slow speeds in a rehabilitation program have been compared. The research literature seems to indicate that strength increases from slow-speed training are relatively specific to the velocity used in training. Conversely, training at faster speeds seems to produce a more generalized increase in torque values at all velocities. Minimal hypertrophy was observed only while training at fast speeds affecting only type II or fast twitch fibers. An increase in neuromuscular efficiency owing to more effective motor unit firing patterns has been domonstrated with slow-speed training. Consequently, during the early 1990s, the value of isokinetic devices for quantifying torque values at functional speeds has been questioned.

Circuit Training

Circuit training is a technique that may be useful to the sports therapist as a means of maintaining or perhaps improving levels of muscular strength or endurance in other parts of the body while the athlete allows for healing and reconditioning of an injured body part. Circuit training utilizes a series of exercise stations that consist of various combinations of weight training, flexibility, calisthenics, and brief aerobic exercises. Circuits may be designed to accomplish many different training goals. With circuit training the athlete moves rapidly from one station to the next, performing whatever exercise is to be done at that station within a specified time period. A typical circuit would consist of 8 to 12 stations, and the entire circuit would be repeated three times.

Circuit training is definitely an effective technique for improving strength and flexibility. Certainly, if the pace or the time interval between stations is rapid and if work load is maintained at a high level of intensity with heart rates at or above target training levels, the cardiorespiratory system may benefit from this circuit. However, there is little research evidence to show that circuit training is very effective in improving cardiorespiratory endurance. It should be and is most often used as a technique for developing and improving muscular strength and endurance.

Plyometric Exercise

Plyometric exercise is a technique that is being increasingly incorporated into later stages of the reconditioning program by the sports therapist. Plyometric training includes specific exercises that encompass a rapid stretch of a muscle eccentrically, followed immediately by a rapid concentric contraction of that muscle for the purpose of facilitating and developing a forceful explosive movement over a short period of time. The greater the stretch put on the muscle from its resting length immediately before the concentric contraction, the greater the resistance the muscle can overcome. Plyometrics emphasize the speed of the eccentric phase. The rate of stretch is more critical than the magnitude of the stretch. An advantage to using plyometric exercises is that they can help to develop eccentric control in dynamic movements.

Plyometric exercises involve hops, bounds, and depth jumping for the lower extremity, and the use of medicine balls and other types of weighted equipment for the upper extremity. Depth jumping is an example of a plyometric exercise in which an individual jumps to the ground from a specified height and then quickly jumps again as soon as ground contact is made.

Plyometrics tend to place a great deal of stress on the musculoskeletal system. The learning and perfection of specific jumping skills and other plyometric exercises must be technically correct and specific to one's age, activity, and physical and skill development.

Open versus Closed Kinetic Chain Exercise

The concept of the kinetic chain deals with the anatomic functional relations that exist in the upper and lower extremities. In a weight-bearing position, the lower extremity kinetic chain involves the transmission of forces between the foot, ankle, lower leg, knee, thigh, and hip. In the upper extremity, when the hand is a weight-bearing surface, forces are transmitted to the wrist, forearm, elbow, upper arm, and shoulder girdle.

An open kinetic chain exists when the foot or hand is not in contact with the ground or some other surface. In a closed kinetic chain, the foot or hand are weight-bearing. Movements of the more proximal

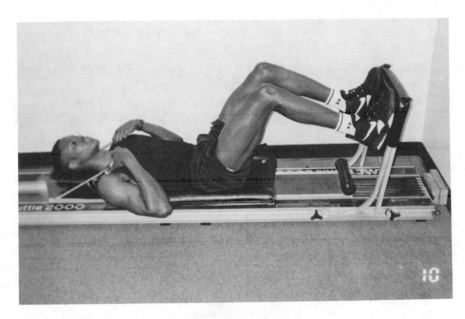

Figure 5.5 *Closed kinetic chain exercises are particularly useful in the rehabilitation of injuries to the lower extremity.*

anatomic segments are affected by these open versus closed kinetic chain positions. For example, the rotational components of the ankle, knee, and hip reverse direction when changing from an open to closed kinetic chain activity. In a closed kinetic chain the forces begin at the ground and work their way up through each joint. Also, in a closed kinetic chain, forces must be absorbed by various tissues and anatomic structures rather than simply dissipating as would occur in an open chain.

In rehabilitation, closed-chain strengthening techniques have become the treatment of choice for many sports therapists. As most sports activities involve some aspect of weight bearing with the foot in contact with the ground, or the hand in a weight-bearing position, closed-chain strengthening activities are more functional than are open-chain activities. Therefore rehabilitative exercises should be incorporated that emphasize strengthening of the entire kinetic chain rather than an isolated body segment (Fig. 5.5).

Maintaining Cardiorespiratory Endurance

Although strength and flexibility are commonly regarded as essential components in any injury rehabilitation program, often relatively little consideration is given to maintaining levels of cardiorespiratory endurance. An athlete spends a considerable amount of time preparing the cardiorespiratory system to handle the increased demands made upon it during a competitive season. When injury occurs and the athlete is forced to miss training time, levels of cardiorespiratory endurance may decrease rapidly. Thus the sports therapist must design or substitute alternative activities that allow the individual to maintain existing levels of fitness during the rehabilitation period (Fig. 5.6).

By definition, cardiorespiratory endurance is the ability to perform whole-body activities for extended periods of time. The cardiorespiratory system provides a means by which oxygen is supplied to the various tissues of the body. Without oxygen the cells within the human body cannot possibly function, and ultimately death will occur. Thus the cardiorespiratory system is the basic life-support system of the body.

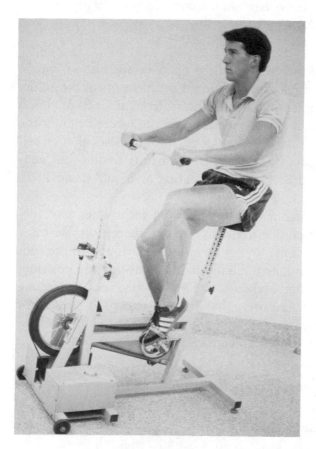

Figure 5.6 *It is critical for the athlete to maintain levels of cardiorespiratory endurance during periods of injury rehabilitation.*

Training Techniques

Several different training techniques through which cardiorespiratory endurance can be maintained may be incorporated into a rehabilitation program. Certainly, a primary consideration for the sports therapist would be whether the injury involves the upper or lower extremity. With injuries that involve the upper extremity, weight-bearing activities such as walking, running, stair climbing, and modified aerobics can be used. However, if the injury is to the lower extremity, alternative non-weight-bearing activities such as swimming or stationary cycling may be necessary.

In a sport such as soccer that requires a considerable amount of running, training using appropriate non-weight-bearing activities will not keep the athlete fit for competition. The only way to achieve such fitness is to engage in functional activities specific to that sport. The goal of the sports therapist in substituting alternative activities during rehabilitation is to maintain a cardiorespiratory endurance base, so that the athlete may quickly regain match fitness once his or her injury has healed.

The principles of the training techniques discussed below can be applied to running, cycling, swimming, stair climbing, or any other activity designed to maintain levels of cardiorespiratory fitness.

Continuous Training

Continuous training involves four considerations: (1) the type of activity, (2) the frequency of the activity, (3) the intensity of the activity, and (4) the duration of the activity.

Type of Activity

The type of activity used in continuous training must be aerobic. Aerobic activities are any type that elevates the heart rate and maintains it at that level for an extended time. Aerobic activities generally involve repetitive, whole-body, large-muscle movements performed over an extended time. Examples of weight-bearing aerobic activities are walking, running, jogging, rope skipping, stepping, aerobic dance exercise, roller blading, and cross-country skiing. Non-weight-bearing aerobic activities include cycling and swimming. The advantage of these aerobic activities as opposed to more intermittent activities such as racquetball, squash, basketball, or tennis, is that aerobic activities are easy to regulate by either speeding up or slowing down the pace. As the intensity of the work load elicits a specific heart rate, these aerobic activities can maintain heart rate at a specified or target level. Intermittent activities involve variable speeds and intensities that cause the heart rate to fluctuate considerably. Although these intermittent activities will improve cardiorespiratory endurance, they are much more difficult to monitor in terms of intensity.

Frequency

To achieve at least minimal improvement in cardiorespiratory endurance, it is necessary for the average person to engage in no less than three sessions per week. A competitive athlete should be prepared to train as often as six times per week. Everyone should rest at least 1 day per week to give damaged tissues a chance to repair themselves.

Intensity

The intensity of the exercise is also a critical factor even though recommendations regarding training intensities vary. This is particularly true in the early stages of training, when the body is forced to make a lot of adjustments to increased work-load demands.

Because heart rate is linearly related to the intensity of the exercise as well as to the rate of oxygen consumption, it becomes a relatively simple process to identify a specific work load (pace) that will make the heart rate plateau at the desired level. By monitoring heart rate, one knows whether the pace is too fast or too slow to get heart rate into a target range.

There are several formulas by which the sports therapist can easily identify a target training heart rate. Exact determination of maximal heart rate involves exercising an athlete at a maximal level and monitoring the heart rate using electrocardiography. This is a difficult process outside a laboratory. However, for both men and women in the population maximal heart rate is thought to be approximately 220 beats per minute. Maximal heart rate is related to age. As one gets older, the maximal heart rate decreases. Thus a relatively simple estimate of maximal heart rate (MHR) would be MHR = 220 − Age. For a 20-year-old athlete, maximal heart rate would be about 200 beats per minute (220 − 20 = 200). If one is interested in working at 70% of one's maximal rate, the target heart rate can be calculated by multiplying 0.7 × (220 − Age). Again using a 20-year-old as an example, target heart rate would be 140 beats per minute (0.7 × [220 − 20] = 140). Another commonly used heart rate (HR) formula that takes into account one's current level of fitness is the Karvonen equation.

Target training HR
    = Resting HR + (0.6[Maximal HR − Resting HR])

Resting heart rate generally falls between 60 and 80 beats per minute. A 20-year-old athlete with a resting pulse of 70 beats per minute, according to the Karvonen equation, would have a target training heart rate of 148 beats per minute (70 + 0.6[200 − 70] = 148). Regardless of the formula used, it should be clear that to achieve minimal improvement in cardiorespiratory endurance, the athlete must train with the heart rate elevated to at least 60% of its maximal rate. The American College of Sports Medicine recommends that for the collegiate athlete, it is more desirable to train in the 60% to 90% range when training continuously. Exercising at a 70% level is considered a moderate level because activity can be continued for a long period of time with little discomfort and still produce a training effect. For a trained individual it is not difficult to sustain a heart rate at the 85% level.

The rate of perceived exertion (RPE) can also be used in addition to monitoring heart rate to indicate exercise intensity. During exercise, individuals are asked to rate subjectively on a numerical scale from 6 to 20 exactly how they feel relative to their level of exertion. More intense exercise that requires a higher level of oxygen consumption and energy expenditure is directly related to higher subjective ratings of perceived exertion. Over a period of time, athletes can be taught to exercise at a specific RPE that relates directly to more objective measures of exercise intensity.

Duration

For minimal improvement to occur, the athlete must participate in at least 20 minutes of continuous activity with the heart rate elevated to its working level. The American College of Sports Medicine recommends 20 to 60 minutes of workout or activity with the heart rate elevated to training levels. Generally, the greater the duration of the workout, the greater the improvement in cardiorespiratory endurance. The competitive athlete should train for at least 45 minutes.

Interval Training

Unlike continuous training, interval training involves activities that are more intermittent. Interval training consists of alternating periods of relatively intense work and active recovery. It allows for performance of much more work at a more intense work load over a longer period of time than if one is working continuously.

For the athlete it is most desirable in continuous training to work at an intensity of about 75% to 80% of maximal heart rate. Obviously, sustaining activity at a higher intensity over a 20-minute period would be difficult. The advantage of interval training is that it allows work at this 80% or higher level for a short period of time, followed by an active period of recovery during which the athlete may be working at only 60% to 70% of maximal heart rate. Thus the intensity of the workout and its duration can be greater than with continuous training.

Most sports are anaerobic, involving short bursts of intense activity followed by a somewhat active recovery period (for example, football, basketball, soccer, or tennis). The interval technique allows training to be more sport-specific during the workout. With interval training the overload principle should be applied, making the training period much more intense.

There are several important considerations in interval training. The training period is the amount of time that continuous activity is actually being performed, and the recovery period is the time between training periods. A set is a group of combined training and recovery periods, and a repetition is the number of training and recovery periods per set. Training time or distance refers to the rate or distance of the training period. The training-recovery ratio indicates a time ratio for training versus recovery.

An example of interval training would be a soccer player running sprints. An interval workout would involve running one set of ten 120-yard sprints in under 18 seconds, with a 45-second walking recovery period between each repetition. During this training session the soccer player's heart rate would probably increase to 85% to 95% of maximal level during the dash and should fall to the 60% to 70% level during the recovery period.

Older athletes should exercise some caution when using interval training as a method for improving cardiorespiratory endurance. The intensity levels attained during the active periods may be too high for the untrained individual.

Reestablishing Proprioception and Neuromuscular Control

Developing a rehabilitation program that incorporates proprioceptively mediated muscular control of joints necessitates an appreciation for the influence of the central nervous system (CNS) on motor activities. Nerve endings relaying sensory information to the CNS, also called afferents, contribute to CNS function and thereby modulate motor or muscle control at three distinct levels. At the spinal level, reflexes mediate reflex splinting during conditions of abnormal stress about the joint and have significant implications for rehabilitation. The muscle spindles play a major role in the control of muscular movement by adjusting activity in the lower motor neurons. The second level of motor control is at the brain stem, where joint afference is relayed to maintain posture and balance of the body. The input to the brain stem about this information emanates from the joint proprioceptors, the vestibular centers in the ears, and from the eyes. The final aspect of motor control includes the highest level of CNS function and is mediated by cognitive awareness of body position and movement. These higher centers initiate and program motor commands for voluntary movements. Movements that are repeated can be stored as central commands and can be performed without continuous reference to consciousness.

With these three levels of motor control in mind, mediated in part by joint and muscle afferents, one can begin to develop rehabilitation activities to address proprioceptive deficiencies. The objectives must be to stimulate the joint and muscle receptors in order to encourage maximum afferent discharge to the respective CNS level. At the spinal level, activities that encourage reflex joint stabilization should be addressed. Such activities include sudden alterations in joint positioning that necessitate reflex muscular stabilization. Balance and postural activities, both with and without visual input, will enhance motor function at the level of the brain stem. Consciously performed joint-positioning activities, especially at joint end ranges, will maximally stimulate the conversion of conscious to unconscious motor programming.

Neuromuscular Control Techniques

Mechanoreceptors located in the joints of the lower extremities are most functionally stimulated when the extremity is positioned in a closed kinetic chain orientation and perpendicular axial loading of the joint is permitted. It is also important that these exercises are performed at various positions throughout the range of joint motion, because of the differences in afferent response that have been observed.

Much attention in sports rehabilitation has been focused on methods to improve proprioception after ankle and knee joint injury in an attempt to decrease the risk of reinjury. Afferent input is altered after joint injury, and it appears to remain altered after joint surgery. The objectives of proprioceptive rehabilitation are to retrain altered afferent pathways, resulting in enhanced sensation of joint movement.

Kinesthetic training begins early in the rehabilitation program, with such simple tasks as balance training and joint repositioning, and becomes increasingly more difficult as the patient progresses. Activities should be structured to address all three of the previously discussed levels of afference-mediated motor control. Once the athlete has reached the functional stage of rehabilitation, the objectives of proprioception training are to refine joint sense awareness in order to initiate muscle reflex stabilization to prevent reinjury. Proprioceptive acuity also plays an important role in the performance of those athletes requiring precision in their movement patterns.

The proprioceptive mechanism comprises both conscious and unconscious pathways. Therefore these exercises should include not only consciously mediated patterned sequences, but also sudden alterations of joint positions that initiate reflex muscle contraction. Kinesthetic training exercises that permit balancing on unstable platforms while enabling the athlete to perform a sport-specific skill integrate both of these neural pathways and maximally stimulate kinesthetic awareness (Fig. 5.7). Therefore kinesthetic exercise progression should begin with balance training and joint position awareness, then progress to highly complex sport-specific activities.

The proprioception component of the rehabilitation program should correspond with the functional progression of the athlete. Proprioception activities can be initiated before weight bearing by having the athlete practice joint repositioning and kinesthetic training using an unstable platform while sitting. Once functional rehabilitation begins kinesthetic activities concentrating on neuromuscular control of the joint should dominate activities. Each phase of the rehabilitation program should attempt to refine kinesthetic acuity that will permit progression to more complex running maneuvers during the ensuing phases of the functional program.

Role of Functional Progressions in Rehabilitation

Sports therapists must adapt rehabilitation to the specific demands required by each sport and playing position. But rehabilitation con-

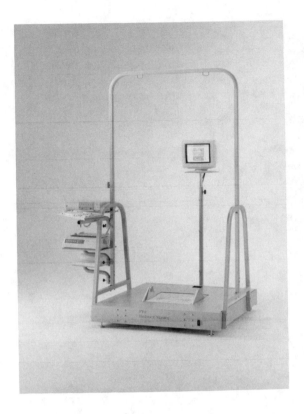

Figure 5.7 *The Kinesthetic Awareness Trainer (KAT) system is an example of a balance device for reestablishing neuromuscular control.*

ducted in a clinical setting cannot predict the effectiveness of the injured part to endure the imposed demands of full competition. For example, a solid, high-velocity tackle cannot be simulated in the clinical setting. The role of the functional progression, then, is to improve and complete the clinical rehabilitation. A functional progression is a succession of activities that simulate actual motor and sport skills, enabling the athlete to acquire or reacquire the skills needed to perform athletic endeavors safely and effectively (Fig. 5.8). The sports therapist breaks down the activities involved in a given sport into individual components. In this way the athlete concentrates on individual parts of the game or activity in a controlled environment before combining them in an uncontrolled environment such as occurs in full competition. The functional progression places stresses and forces on each body system in a well-planned, positive, and progressive fashion, ultimately improving the athlete's overall ability to meet the demands placed upon him or her in daily activities as well as in sports competition. The functional progression is indicated because tissues not placed under performance-level stresses do not adapt to the sudden return of such stresses with the resumption of full

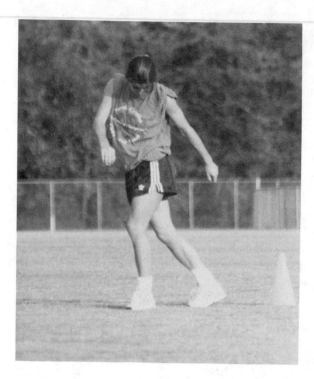

Figure 5.8 *Functional progressions involve breaking sport activities into component parts and gradually increasing the load and intensity of the activity.*

activity. Thus the functional progression is integrated into the normal rehabilitation scheme, as one component of exercise therapy, rather than replacing traditional rehabilitation altogether.

Generally, rehabilitation of sport-related injuries has two goals. One is minimizing further trauma to injured structures and safely and quickly returning the injured athlete to previous levels of competition. The other rehabilitation goal is divided into three main stages: immediate, short-term, and long-term goals. The immediate goal begins at the time of injury and involves the treatment or management of the injury. This includes protection from further injury, restricted activity, and controls to minimize pain and swelling. The short-term goal deals with the healing process, enabling the symptoms and level of dysfunction to subside. Also during this stage, uninvolved body parts can be exercised to maintain normal function and fitness levels. The long-term goal overlaps the short-term goal and involves progression to a point of full return to activity. Once the athlete meets criteria to return to controlled activity, exercise therapy is begun. The functional progression serves as a component of exercise therapy to help the athlete meet the preset criteria for return to play.

Benefits of Using Functional Progressions

Functional progressions provide both physical and psychologic benefits to the injured athlete. Strength, endurance, mobility, flexibility, relaxation, coordination, and skill can be restored. At the same time the functional stability of the joint can be assessed, providing the physical benefits. Psychologically, the progression can reduce the feelings of anxiety, apprehension, and deprivation commonly observed in the injured athlete.

Rehabilitation Tools

Therapeutic Modalities

Therapeutic modalities, when used appropriately, can be extremely useful tools in the rehabilitation of the injured athlete. As with any other tool, their effectiveness is limited by the knowledge, skill, and experience of the person using them. For the sports therapist, decisions regarding how and when a modality may best be employed should be based on a combination of theoretical knowledge and practical experience. Modalities should not be used at random, nor should their use be based on what has been done in the past. Rather, consideration must always be given to what should work best in a specific clinical situation.

In any program of rehabilitation, modalities should be used primarily as adjuncts to therapeutic exercise and certainly not at the exclusion of range-of-motion and strengthening exercises. There are many different approaches and ideas regarding the use of modalities in injury rehabilitation. Therefore no "cookbook" exists for modality use. Rather, sports therapists should make their own decisions from the options in a given clinical situation about which modality will be most effective.

Among the therapeutic modalities most typically used by sports therapists are electrical stimulating currents, electromyographic biofeedback, shortwave and microwave diathermy, infrared, low-power laser, ultrasound, and intermittent compression (Fig. 5.9).

Electrical Stimulating Currents

Most stimulators have the flexibility to alter the frequency output of the device to elicit a desired physiologic response. The electrical stimulating currents are capable of (1) pain modulation either through transcutaneous electrical nerve stimulation (TENS) at high

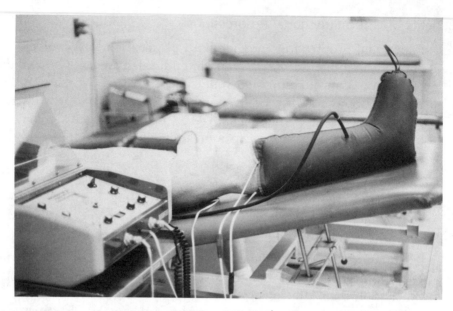

Figure 5.9 *Therapeutic modalities should be used in rehabilitation as adjuncts to other types of therapeutic exercise.*

frequencies, or through production of β-endorphin at lower frequencies (electroacutherapy); (2) producing muscle contraction and relaxation or tetany depending on the type of current (alternating or direct) and frequency (Russian currents); (3) facilitating soft tissue and bone healing through the use of low intensity stimulation (LIS); and (4) producing a net movement of ions through the use of continuous direct current and thus eliciting a chemical change in the tissues (iontophoresis).

Electromyographic Biofeedback

Electromyographic biofeedback is a therapeutic procedure that uses electronic or electromechanical instruments to accurately measure, process, and return reinforcing information via auditory or visual signals. In sports medicine, it is used to help the athlete develop greater voluntary control in terms of either neuromuscular relaxation or muscle reeducation following injury.

Shortwave and Microwave Diathermy

The diathermies are considered to be high-frequency currents because they have more than a million cycles per second. When impulses of such a short duration come in contact with human tissue, there is not sufficient time for ion movement to take place. Consequently there is no stimulation of either motor or sensory nerves. The energy of this rapidly vibrating electrical current produces heat as it passes through tissue cells, resulting in a temperature increase. Shortwave diathermy may be either continuous or pulsed. Both continuous shortwave and microwave diathermy are used primarily for their thermal effects, while pulsed shortwave is used for its nonthermal effects.

Infrared Modalities

The largest number of modalities used by sports therapists may be collectively classified as infrared modalities. Cold packs, hydrocollator packs, whirlpools, paraffin baths, and contrast baths are all infrared modalities. The infrared modalities are used to produce a local and occasionally a generalized heating or cooling of the superficial tissues. The infrared modalities may also elicit either increases or decreases in circulation depending on whether heat or cold is used. They are also known to have analgesic effects as a result of stimulation of sensory cutaneous nerve endings.

Low-Power Laser

The low-power laser is certainly the newest modality used by the sports therapist. The low-power or cold laser produces little or no thermal effects but seems to have a clinical effect on soft tissue and fracture healing as well as pain management through stimulation of acupuncture and trigger points. Two types of low-power lasers are used by sports therapists: the helium-neon (HeNe) laser and the gallium-arsenide (GaAs) laser.

Ultrasound

Along with the electrical stimulating currents and the infrared modalities, ultrasound is one of the most widely used treatment modalities. Ultrasound is a mechanical vibration, a sound wave, produced and transformed from high-frequency electrical energy. Therapeutic ultrasound has traditionally been used to increase tissue temperature through thermal physiologic effects. However, it is also capable of enhancing healing at the cellular level as a result of its nonthermal physiologic effects.

Intermittent Compression

Edema that accumulates following injury or surgery can be effectively managed using intermittent compression. This treatment, along with external elastic supports, elevation, weight bearing, and exercise, will help reverse the edema and prevent its reaccumulation. Some intermittent compression units also incorporate cold therapy. These combination units appear to be more effective in reducing edema than compression alone.

Treatment parameters are better understood from clinic empiricism than from research studies. While attempting to use the physiologic principles of edema accumulation and reduction to create minimum and maximum values, one should follow patient comfort as the primary guide for specific manipulations of on-off times, pressure, and total treatment time.

Joint Mobilization Techniques

The techniques of joint mobilization are used to improve joint mobility or to decrease joint pain by restoring accessory movements to the joint and thus allowing full, nonrestricted, pain-free range of motion. Mobilization techniques may be used to attain a variety of treatment goals: reducing pain; decreasing muscle guarding; stretching or lengthening tissue surrounding a joint, in particular capsular and ligamentous tissue; reflexogenic effects that either inhibit or facilitate muscle tone or stretch reflex; and proprioceptive effects to improve postural and kinesthetic awareness.

Basically two types of movement govern motion about a joint. Perhaps the better known of the two types are the physiologic movements that result from an active muscle contraction that moves an extremity through traditional cardinal planes including flexion, extension, abduction, adduction, and rotation. The second type is called accessory motion. Accessory motion refers to the manner in which one articulating joint surface moves relative to another. Accessory motions are also referred to as joint arthrokinematics, which include spin, roll, and glide.

Movement throughout a range of motion can be quantified with various measurement techniques. Physiologic movement is measured with a goniometer and comprises the major portion of the range. Accessory motion is expressed in millimeters, although precise measurement is difficult.

Accessory movements may be hypomobile, normal, or hypermobile. Each joint has a range-of-motion continuum with an anatomic limit to motion that is determined by both bony arrangement and surrounding soft tissue (Fig. 5.10). In a hypomobile joint, motion stops at some point referred to as a pathologic point of

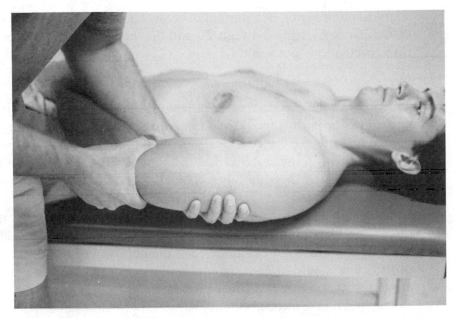

Figure 5.10 *Joint mobilization requires a therapist with special skills and knowledge in that area.*

limitation, short of the anatomic limit, because of pain, spasm, or tissue resistance.

A hypermobile joint moves beyond its anatomic limit because of laxity in the surrounding structures. A hypomobile joint should respond well to techniques of mobilization and traction. A hypermobile joint should be treated with strengthening exercises, stability exercises, and, if indicated, taping, splinting, or bracing.

Treatment techniques designed to improve accessory movement are generally small-amplitude movements, the amplitude being the distance that the joint is moved passively within its total range. Mobilization techniques utilize these small-amplitude oscillating motions that glide or slide one of the articulating joint surfaces in an appropriate direction within a specific part of the range.

Mobilization should be done with both the athlete and the sports therapist positioned in a comfortable and relaxed manner. The sports therapist should mobilize one joint at a time. The joint should be stabilized as near one articulating surface as possible, while the other segment is moved with a firm, confident grasp. Joints that are stiff or hypomobile and have restricted movement should be treated three to four times per week, alternating days with active motion exercise.

Typical mobilization of a joint may involve a series of three to six sets of oscillations lasting between 20 and 60 seconds each, with one to three oscillations per second.

Traction

Traction may be used to treat a variety of joint problems either in the extremities or in the cervical and lumbar spine. Traction may be done manually or using a mechanical device. Manual traction is usually combined with joint mobilization techniques either to decrease pain or to reduce joint hypomobility. Traction stretches the joint capsule and increases the space between the articulating surfaces, thus enhancing gliding oscillations. Mechanical traction devices are most often used with problems of the cervical or lumbar spine. The effect of traction on each system involved in the complex anatomic makeup of the spine should be considered when selecting traction as a part of a therapeutic treatment plan (Fig. 5.11).

The traction protocol should be set up to manage a particular problem rather than applied in the same manner regardless of the patient or pathology. Traction is a flexible modality with an infinite number of variations available. This flexibility should allow sports

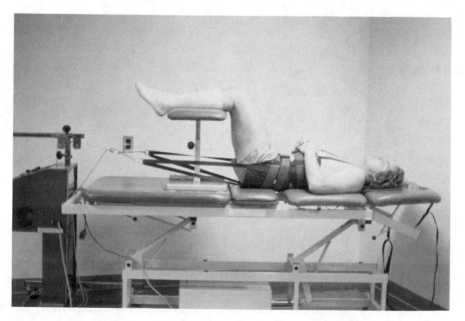

Figure 5.11 *Traction techniques may be used to treat both pain and hypomobility in a joint.*

therapists to adjust their protocols to match the patient's symptoms and diagnosis.

Traction is capable of producing a separation of vertebral bodies; a centripetal force on the soft tissues surrounding the vertebrae; a mobilization of vertebral joints; a change in proprioceptive discharge of the spinal complex; a stretch of connective tissue; a stretch of muscle tissue; an improvement in arterial, venous, and lymphatic flow; and a lessening of the compressive effects of posture. Any of these effects can change the symptoms of the patient under treatment and help to normalize the patient's lumbar or cervical spine.

Proprioceptive Neuromuscular Facilitation

Proprioceptive neuromuscular facilitation (PNF) is an approach to therapeutic exercise based on the principles of functional human anatomy and neurophysiology. It utilizes proprioceptive, cutaneous, and auditory input to produce functional improvement in motor output and can be a vital element in the rehabilitation process of many sports-related injuries. As a positive approach to injury rehabilitation, PNF is aimed at what the patient can do physically within the limitations of the injury. It is perhaps best utilized for decreasing deficiencies in strength, flexibility, and coordination in response to demands that are placed on the neuromuscular systems.

The PNF approach is holistic, integrating sensory, motor, and psychological aspects of a rehabilitation program. It incorporates reflex activities from the spinal levels and upward, either inhibiting or facilitating them as appropriate.

The principles and techniques of PNF described here are based primarily on the neurophysiologic mechanisms involving the stretch reflex. Impulses transmitted from the peripheral stretch receptors via the afferent system and the CNS have the strongest influence on the motor neurons supplying the muscles. Therefore the sports therapist should be able to modify the input from the peripheral receptors and thus influence the excitability of the motor neurons. The discharge of motor neurons can be facilitated by peripheral stimulation and results in increased muscle tone or strength of voluntary contraction. Conversely, motor neurons can be inhibited by peripheral stimulation, which causes afferent impulses to make contact with inhibitory neurons, thus resulting in muscle relaxation and allowing for stretching of the muscle. Thus PNF techniques may be used in a rehabilitation program either for strengthening or support of a particular agonistic muscle group or for stretching or inhibition of the antagonistic group. The choice of a specific technique depends on the deficits of a particular patient. Specific techniques or combinations of techniques should be selected on the basis of the patient's problem.

Therapeutic Massage

Massage is mechanical stimulation of tissues by means of rhythmically applied pressure and stretching (Fig. 5.12). Over the years many claims have been made relative to the therapeutic benefits of massage in the athletic population, although few are based on well-controlled and well-designed studies. Athletes have used massage to increase flexibility and coordination as well as to increase their pain threshold; to decrease neuromuscular excitability in the muscle being massaged; to stimulate circulation, thus improving energy transport to the muscle; to facilitate healing and restore joint mobility; and to remove lactic acid, thus alleviating muscle cramps. Conclusive evidence of the efficacy of massage as an ergogenic aid in the athletic population is lacking.

How these effects may be accomplished is determined by the specific approaches used with massage techniques and how they are applied. Generally the effects of massage may be either reflexive or mechanical. The effect of massage on the nervous system will differ greatly according to the method used, the pressure exerted, and the duration of applications. Through the reflex mechanism, sedation is induced. Slow, gentle, rhythmical, and superficial effleurage may relieve tension and soothe, rendering the muscles more relaxed. This indicates an effect on sensory and motor nerves locally and some CNS

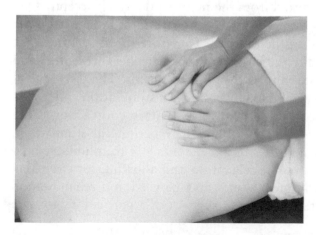

Figure 5.12 *Massage techniques may be useful for relaxation, for stimulating circulation, for pain modulation, or for soft tissue adhesion that restricts motion.*

response. The mechanical approach seeks to make mechanical or histologic changes in myofascial structures through direct force applied superficially.

Many massage techniques have been described. Most rely heavily on theoretical assumptions and have not been researched in a scientific manner. However, many athletes report positive effects from massage, and it can be a useful adjunct to rehabilitation in selected cases. A few techniques will be described.

Hoffa Massage

Hoffa massage is essentially the classic massage technique that uses a variety of superficial strokes including effleurage, petrissage, tapotment, and vibration. Although some clinicians consider this technique to be mechanical, the strokes may be lighter and more superficial, thus making them more reflexive in nature. This technique opens the door for more mechanical techniques directed toward underlying tissues.

Friction Massage

Friction massage may be used to affect musculoskeletal structures of ligament, tendon, and muscle to provide therapeutic movement over a small area. The purposes for friction movements are to loosen adherent fibrous tissue (scar), aid in the absorption of local edema or effusions, and reduce local muscular spasm. Inflammation around joints is softened and more readily broken down so that the formation of adhesions is prevented. Another purpose is to provide deep pressure over trigger points to produce reflex effects. This technique is performed by the tips of the fingers, the thumb, or the heel of the hand, according to the area to be covered, making small circular movements. The superficial tissues are moved over the underlying structures by keeping the hand or fingers in firm contact with the skin.

Acupressure and Trigger Point Massage

Acupressure is a type of massage based on the ancient Chinese art of acupuncture. According to acupuncture theory, stimulation of specific points through needling can dramatically reduce pain in areas of the body known to be associated with a particular point. In Western medicine, the counterpart of the acupuncture point is the trigger point. Trigger points may be found in skeletal muscle and tendons, in myofascia, in ligaments and capsules surrounding joints, in periosteum, and in the skin. Trigger points become painful because of some trauma to the muscle, occurring either from direct trauma or from overuse, which results in an inflammatory response. With both acupuncture and trigger point massage, pain is usually referred to areas that follow a specific pattern associated with a particular point. Stimulation of these points through massage has been demonstrated to result in a relief of pain.

Myofascial Release

Myofascial release refers to a group of techniques used for the purpose of relieving soft tissue from the abnormal grip of tight fascia. It is essentially a form of stretching that has been reported to have significant impact in treating a variety of conditions. Some specialized training is necessary for the sports therapist to understand specific techniques of myofascial release in addition to an in-depth understanding of the fascial system.

Myofascial release has also been referred to as soft tissue mobilization although technically all forms of massage involve mobilization of soft tissue. Soft tissue mobilization should not be confused with joint mobilization although the two are closely related.

Myofascial treatment is based on localizing the restriction and moving into the direction of the restriction regardless of whether that follows the arthrokinematics of a nearby joint. Thus myofascial manipulation is considerably more subjective and relies heavily on the experience of the clinician.

Aquatic Therapy

In the past decade, widespread interest has developed in the area of aquatic therapy. It has rapidly become a popular rehabilitation technique among sports therapists. Aquatic therapy is beneficial in the treatment of everything from orthopedic injuries to spinal cord damage, chronic pain, cerebral palsy, multiple sclerosis, and many other conditions, making it useful in a variety of settings.

Aquatic therapy is believed to be successful because it lowers pain levels by decreasing joint compression forces. The perception of weightlessness experienced in the water seems to eliminate or drastically reduce the body's protective muscular guarding. This effect results in decreased muscular spasm and pain, which may carry over into the patient's daily functional activities. The primary goal of aquatic therapy is to teach the athlete how to use water as a modality for improving movement and fitness (Fig. 5.13). Then, along with other therapeutic modalities and treatments, aquatic therapy can

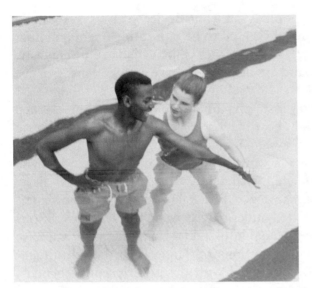

Figure 5.13 *Aquatic therapy can be used to exercise an injured part when weight bearing may exacerbate the injury.*

become one more link in the athlete's recovery chain. An aquatic therapy program offers many advantages. Physiologically, aquatic therapy is similar to land exercises in that blood supply, muscle temperature, metabolism, oxygen demand, and oxygen production increase just as they do in land exercises. The characteristics that are making aquatic therapy popular are those that separate it from traditional land exercises. Very fine gradation of exercise can be manipulated by utilizing combinations of the different resistive forces. For instance, when using weights on land, the athlete is limited to the equipment available. If the 10-pound dumbbell is too heavy, yet the 5-pound dumbbell is too light, there is no middle ground. With aquatic therapy, however, extremely small gradations of intensity can be controlled by changing the body positioning or the equipment being used. Through water exercises even persons with minimal muscle contraction capabilities can do work and see improvement when they were unable to do so on land.

A further advantage of aquatic therapy concerns weight-bearing principles. The patient can safely begin locomotor activities earlier in the rehabilitation process following a lower extremity injury by using the buoyant force to decrease the apparent weight and compressive forces. This advantage is of great importance to the athletic population in particular. Through careful use of Archimedes' principle, a gradual increase in the percentage of weight bearing can be undertaken. Initially, the athlete would begin non-weight-bearing exercise in the deep end of the pool. A buoyant device such as a specially designed waterski vest might be used to help the athlete remain afloat for the desired exercises. If such a device is unavailable, empty plastic milk jugs held in each hand are also an effective and very inexpensive method of flotation.

Once therapy has progressed the athlete could move to neck-deep water to begin light weight bearing. The percentage of weight bearing is gradually increased by systematically moving the athlete to more shallow water. Even when in waist-deep water, both male and female athletes are only bearing approximately 50% of their total body weight. By placing a sinkable bench or chair in the shallow water, step-ups can then be initiated under partial-weight-bearing conditions long before the athlete is capable of performing the same exercise under full-weight-bearing conditions on land. Thus the advantages of low weight bearing are coupled with the proprioceptive benefits of closed kinetic chain exercise, making an excellent functional rehabilitation activity.

Another advantage of aquatic therapy is increased range of motion as the warmth of the water helps to induce muscular relaxation. The proprioceptive stimulation from the water may also serve as a gating mechanism in decreasing pain. Muscular strengthening and reeducation can also be accomplished in the aquatic environment. Progressive resistance exercises can gradually be made more difficult as the athlete's strength increases. The water also serves as an accommodating resistance medium. Therefore the muscles are maximally stressed as the athlete works through the full range of motion available, helping to facilitate strength gains. However, the extent of the gains depends on the effort exerted by the athlete and is not easily measured.

Strength gains through aquatic exercise are also brought about by the increased energy needs of the body when working in an aquatic environment. Studies have shown that aquatic exercise requires a higher energy expenditure than the same exercise performed on land. The athlete not only has to perform the activity, but also must maintain a level of buoyancy and overcome the resistive forces of the water. The energy cost for running in water, for example, is four times greater than that for running the same distance on land.

Psychologically, aquatic therapy increases confidence as the athlete experiences increased success at locomotor, stretching, or strengthening activities in the water. Tension and anxiety are decreased, and the athlete's morale increases as well as postexercise vigor.

Full Return to Activity

Allowing the athlete to return to play at full participation is a difficult decision that requires a complete evaluation of the athlete's condition, including objective observations as well as subjective evaluation. The sports therapist should feel that the athlete is ready both physically and mentally before allowing a return to play. Return to activity should not be attempted too soon in order to avoid exacerbation of the injury, which may interfere with healing and result in longer, more painful recovery or perhaps reinjury. In a sports medicine setting, injured athletes are rarely completely healed when they return to full competition. Hence the athlete is certainly susceptible to further injury. In order to release an athlete to full participation, a few criteria should be met:

1. Physician's release
2. Freedom from pain
3. No swelling
4. Normal range of motion
5. Normal strength (in reference to opposite extremity)
6. Appropriate functional testing completed with no adverse reactions

Suggested Readings

Arnheim D, Prentice WE. Principles of athletic training. St. Louis: CV Mosby, 1993.

Astrand PO, Rodahl K. Textbook of work physiology. New York: McGraw-Hill, 1986.

Bandy W, et al. Adaptation of skeletal muscle to resistance training. J Orthop Sports Phys Ther 1992;12(6):248–255.

Barak T, Rosen E, Sofer R. Mobility: passive orthopedic manual therapy. In: Gould J, Davies G, eds. Orthopedic and sports physical therapy. St. Louis: CV Mosby, 1990;212–224.

Barrack RL, Skinner HB, Brunet ME. Proprioception in the anterior cruciate deficient knee. Am J Sports Med 1989;17:1–6.

Cantu RI, Grodin AJ. Myofascial manipulation: theory and clinical applications. Gaithersburg, MD: Aspen Publications, 1992.

Cookson J, Kent B. Orthopedic manual therapy: an overview. Part I: the extremities. Phys Ther 1979;59:136.

Croce P, Greg J. Keeping fit when injured. Clin Sports Med 1991; 10(1):181–195.

Davis M. Rehabilitation of sports injuries: a practical approach. In: Bernhardt D, ed. Sports physical therapy. Philadelphia: Churchill Livingstone, 1986; 155–171.

Kaltenborn F. Mobilization of the extremity joints: examination and basic treatment techniques. Norway: Olaf Norlis Bokhandel, 1980.

Kegerreis S. The construction and implementation of functional progressions as a component of athletic rehabilitation. J Orthop Sports Phys Ther 1983;63(4):14–19.

Knight KL. Cryotherapy: theory, technique and physiology. Chattanooga, TN: Chattanooga Corporation, 1985.

Kolb ME. Principles of underwater exercise. Phys Ther Rev 1957;27(6):361–364.

Lephart S, Kocher M, Fu F. Proprioception following ACL reconstruction. J Sports Rehab 1992;1:186–196.

Prentice WE. A comparison of static and PNF stretching for improvement of hip joint flexibility. Athletic Training 1983;18(1):56–61.

Prentice WE. Rehabilitation techniques in sports medicine. St. Louis: CV Mosby, 1994.

Prentice WE, Kooima E. The use of PNF techniques in rehabilitation of sport-related injury. Athletic Training 1986;21(1):26–31.

Sanders M. Weight training and conditioning. In: Sanders B, ed. Sports physical therapy. Norwalk, CT: Appleton Lange, 1990;239–249.

PART TWO

Regional Injuries

CHAPTER 6

Neck Injuries

Eugene L. Kastelberg, Jr., Walton W. Curl, D. Montgomery Hunter, and David F. Martin

In 1975, the National Football League reported data from two 5-year surveys of head and neck injuries. From 1959 to 1963, there had been 56 fractures or dislocations (a rate of 1.4 per 100,000 athletes) and 30 injuries leading to quadriplegia, which indicates paralysis involving all four extremities (a rate of 0.7 per 100,000 athletes). In the period 1971 to 1975, these numbers had increased to 259 fractures or dislocations (a rate of 4.1 per 100,000 athletes) and 99 injuries leading to quadriplegia (a rate of 1.58 per 100,000 athletes). During that time, it had been legal to use one's helmet as an instrument for tackling ("spearing"); in fact, the technique had been taught to players as part of their training. In 1976, the National Collegiate Athletic Association ruled that no player should intentionally strike another with the crown or top of his helmet or use the helmet to butt or ram; thus "spearing" was outlawed. The year before this rule became effective, there had been 6.5 injuries per 100,000 athletes in high school games and 29.3 injuries per 100,000 athletes in college games. Eight years after this rule became effective, there were only 1.9 injuries per 100,000 athletes in high school and only 6.7 injuries per 100,000 athletes in college.

The cervical neck and spine injuries that occur in current sports competitions are still a challenge to the sports medicine provider, ranging, as they do, from simple strains to catastrophic injuries that can lead to permanent disability. In this chapter, we will discuss the more common soft tissue injuries of the neck, their treatment, and the criteria for the athletes' return to play.

Anatomy

The bony portion of the cervical spine is composed of seven vertebrae: numbered C1 through C7; C1, C2, and C7 are specialized vertebrae; C3–C6 are more typical of the lower vertebrae. Vertebrae C2 through C7 are separated by cartilaginous disks (Fig. 6.1).

The C1 and C2 vertebrae make up the atlanto-axial complex (Fig. 6.2). C1, or the atlas, has an anterior bony ridge, but lacks a body; instead, it is a ring consisting of an anterior and a posterior arch connected by two lateral facets. Its concave superior facets form a joint with the occipital condyles to allow flexion and extension of the head. The inferior facets face downward to form a joint with the superior facets of C2 (Fig. 6.3).

The C2 vertebra, or the axis, has a body, which allows pivoting of C1 for rotational movement of the head. This body—the odontoid process, or dens—is an important structure for both stability and movement.

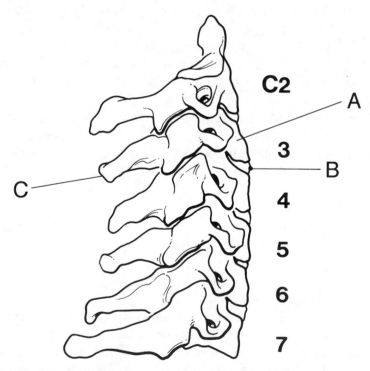

Figure 6.1 *The cervical spine from C2 to C7. Each vertebral body (A) is separated by a cervical disk (B) whereas spinous processes (C) are connected with interspinous ligaments.*

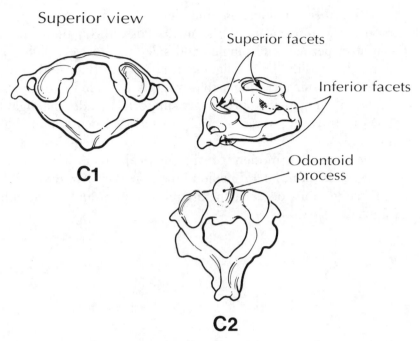

Figure 6.2 *C1 and C2 make up the atlanto-axial complex.*

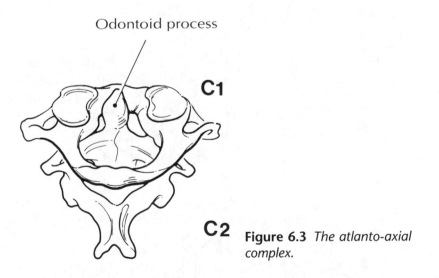

Figure 6.3 *The atlanto-axial complex.*

Vertebrae C3 through C6 are of similar configuration, with small oval bodies that are concave on the superior surface and convex on the inferior surface.

C7 is a transitional vertebra. In contrast to the C3–C6 vertebrae, it has a longer spinous process, a broader body, and a larger and more posterior transverse process.

A number of muscles and ligaments help to support and control the movement of the head. Posteriorly, these include the paired trapezius, semispinalis, and splenius muscles, each separated along the midline by the ligamentum nuchae (Fig. 6.4). Anteriorly, scalene and sternocleidomastoid muscles provide important support (Fig. 6.5). Ligaments providing support include the ligamentum flavum and the anterior and posterior longitudinal ligaments (Fig. 6.6).

The range of motion of the cervical spine includes forward flexion-extension, lateral flexion, and rotation. Approximately 50% of these motions occur at the atlanto-occipital and the atlanto-axial joints.

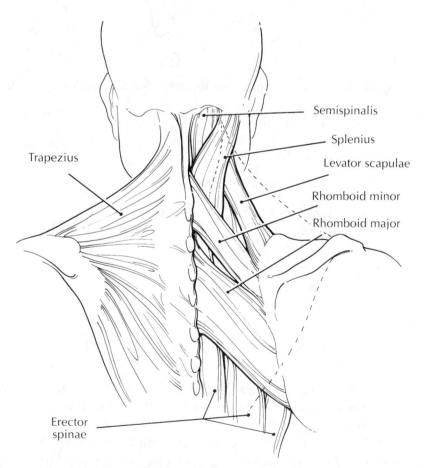

Figure 6.4 *The major muscles along the posterior aspect of the cervical spine.*

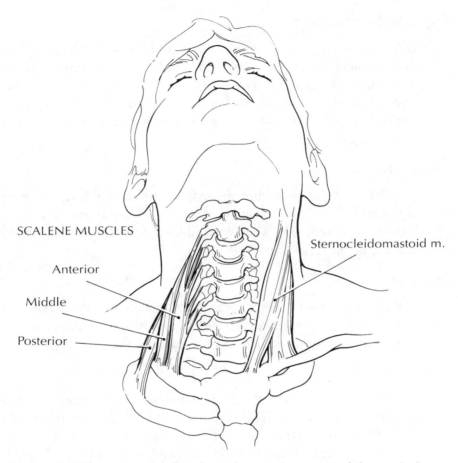

Figure 6.5 *The major muscles along the anterior aspect of the cervical spine.*

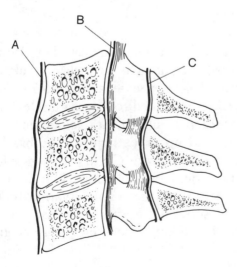

Figure 6.6 *The anterior (A) and posterior (B) longitudinal ligaments as well as the ligamentum flavum (C) are major supporting ligaments of the cervical spine.*

Physical Examination

Before examination, the caregiver should obtain a detailed history that includes onset of symptoms, mechanism of injury, previous injuries, and all symptoms experienced by the athlete since the injury. The physical examination can be divided into five categories: inspection, palpation, range of motion, neurologic examination, and special tests.

Inspection

Inspection begins when the athlete first enters the room. The posture of the athlete and any deviation of the head from the neutral position should be noted. The skin is examined for ecchymosis, swelling, masses, or previous scars.

Palpation

The examiner must palpate the anterior, posterior, and lateral aspects of the neck. Any tenderness, swelling, or masses should be noted. Palpation is carried out laterally to the shoulder.

Range of Motion

The range of motion of the neck includes flexion, extension, lateral bending, and rotation. The athlete should be able to touch chin to chest (flexion) and to look at the ceiling (extension). With lateral bending, the head should be able to bend at least to a 45° angle to each shoulder. With rotation, the athlete's chin is almost in line with the shoulder.

Neurologic Examination

The neurologic examination includes not only the neck, but also the upper extremity and the upper back region. The intrinsic musculature of the neck is tested with resisted flexion, extension, rotation, and lateral bending. The lateral back is examined to assess muscle development, symmetry, and proper scapular movement. Next attention is directed at the brachial plexus and upper extremity. The brachial plexus is made up of the cervical roots from C5 to T1. It provides both sensory and motor function to the upper extremity. It not only supplies the upper extremity, but also supplies innervation to the rhomboids, suprascapular, and serratus anterior muscles. With a detailed examination of the upper extremity, including sensory, motor, and reflex components, an injury to the plexus can be located precisely.

Special Tests

Several special tests can be done during the physical examination that can give insight into the potential cause of the pain. These include the distraction and compression test as well as Adson's test.

The distraction test also helps to detect narrowing of the neural foramen with impingement of the exiting nerve root. The examiner lifts the head, placing one hand under the athlete's chin and the other on the occiput. The examiner then gradually applies pressure to remove the weight of the head from the neck. A positive test is one in which the symptoms, in particular arm pain, are relieved.

The compression test is basically the opposite of the distraction test. Rather than relieving the weight on the cervical spine, the examiner applies pressure on the head to compress the cervical spine. If neural foramen or facet joint pathology or muscle spasms exist, the athlete will experience increased pain. Furthermore, if this pain is reproduced into the upper extremity, the exact neurologic level of injury may be discovered.

If the athlete's subcalvian artery is compressed by an extra cervical rib or by tightened scalenus muscle, circulation and neural structures to the upper extremity can be impaired. Adson's test is used to determine the compression of the vascular supply to the arm.

Adson's test is performed by taking the radial pulse of the patient at the wrist and abducting, extending, and externally rotating the arm. The examiner instructs the athlete to take a deep breath, hold it, and turn his or her head toward the arm being tested. The test is positive if a marked diminution or absence of the radial pulse is found.

Injuries

Quadriplegia

The most catastrophic cervical spine injury is a fracture dislocation resulting in complete paralysis of all extremities or quadriplegia. The most common mechanism for this injury is axial loading due to the application of a direct force to the crown of the head. This type of injury can occur in a number of sports including football, diving, equestrian events, and gymnastics. If this injury is suspected, proper emergency techniques should be used. Each person on the medical team should know the role he or she plays when such an injury occurs and frequent practice sessions are advised. Early management and stabilization of these injuries can have a significant effect on final outcomes.

Preparation

Preparation to manage an athlete with a cervical spine injury begins long before the athlete reaches the practice or playing field. The sports medicine team must be prepared to act quickly and efficiently. This requires a total team effort and a well-thought-out plan of action, with each team member having designated roles and assignments. This emergency plan of action should be written out, complete with names and assigned roles. Once the plan is developed and in place, proper preparation requires education, equipment availability, and experience gained through practice. Education includes not only instructing the sports medicine staff in their roles, but also educating the coaching staff and players. Specifically, the coaches and athletes should be advised never to help or assist an injured player up off the playing field. A player who cannot remove himself from the field requires the assistance of the sports medicine team. Also, teammates and coaches should be advised never to unbuckle a chin strap or remove the helmet from an injured player; this unnecessary movement to the head and neck could worsen an underlying neck injury. For the same reason, coaches and trainers should avoid the use of ammonia or other noxious stimuli to help arouse a player who has received a blow to the head. The sudden jerking movement of the head, in response to the noxious stimuli, could cause permanent damage to an underlying injured spinal cord.

Equipment availability is critical. Proper emergency equipment must be on-site and easily accessible at any practice, game, or event at which an injury may occur. In an emergency, precious seconds cannot be wasted searching for equipment. The following list includes the minimal recommended equipment that should be on hand.

1. Telecommunications—cellular telephone or immediate phone access to call emergency services.
2. Long spine board.
3. Rigid cervical collar.
4. Sandbags to secure the head and neck.

5. An instrument to remove the face mask of a helmet—sharp-nosed pruning shears or snips, an electric screw driver, or the "trainer's angel" (a pair of shears with razor blades as cutting edges).
6. A pocket mask for cardiopulmonary resuscitation (CPR).
7. Basic emergency airway equipment including suction—personnel must be properly trained in the use of oral airways and bag mask setup.

Experience gained from practice is the third essential component of preparation. Every member of the sports medicine team should have a designated role. Drills should be practiced regularly, at least twice a year, to ensure all know their roles and can demonstrate proficiency in meeting their responsibilities.

General Approach

The following guidelines describe the general approach for the neck-injured athlete. Special precautions may have to be added in the case of loss of consciousness.

1. Quickly assess the athlete's level of consciousness. The AVPU scale provides a good initial guideline (A = alert and oriented; V = responsive to verbal stimuli; P = responsive to painful stimuli; U = unresponsive).

2. Regardless of the patient's level of consciousness the ABCDs (airway, breathing, circulation, and disability) of emergency care must be attended first. An obstructed airway must be cleared. If breathing or pulse is absent, CPR should be initiated.

3. Assume underlying brain or cervical spine injury. Remember that 10% of unconscious patients have an underlying cervical spine injury. Any alteration in the level of consciousness can also alter the athlete's perception of pain; therefore the response to questions or palpation of the cervical spine may not be reliable. Assess the disability by examining motor and sensory function in all extremities.

4. If a neck injury is suspected, apply in-line neutral stabilization of the head and neck. (a) If the athlete's head and neck are not in neutral alignment, maintain stabilization in the position until the athlete can be positioned in the face-up position on a spine board. (b) The member of the team stabilizing the head and neck must be prepared to stay with the athlete through the duration of acute care.

5. Position the athlete in the face-up position on the spine board. (a) This requires specialized and choreographed training in the log roll technique to maintain cervical spine immobilization. This requires four or five members of the sports medicine team, all of which must have exhibited proficiency in this maneuver. Otherwise, this should not be attempted until appropriately trained personnel are available. (b) The person controlling the head and neck directs all commands and actions. (c) For the athlete in the prone position, log roll onto the spine board. Raise the spine board at an angle to meet the patient and lower both gently to the ground. (d) For the athlete in the supine position, log roll onto the patient's left side, place the spine board against the patient, and lower both gently to the ground. (e) Secure in-line neutral positioning of the head and neck by applying sand bags against the side of the head or by strapping or taping across the helmet to the spine board. (f) Secure the body straps of the spine board to ensure stability during transport. Remove the face mask from the athlete's helmet to allow access to the airway. *Do not remove the helmet.* Even if the athlete is awake and alert and seemingly doing well, the face mask should be removed to allow rapid access to the airway in the event of a sudden change in mental status.

6. Reassess level of consciousness and other injuries.

7. Prepare to transport the athlete to the hospital. (a) The trainer at the head of the athlete should stay with the athlete. (b) Reassess the ABCDs every 5 minutes during transport. (c) Contact with the parents or guardian should be made to inform them of the injury and of the location of the hospital.

The above only describes a general approach. Again, it should be emphasized that this requires special training and equipment to avoid worsening of these potentially life-threatening injuries.

Acute Torticollis

Acute torticollis (wry neck) consists of the sudden onset of neck pain with stiffness and usually lateral flexion. There may have been a preceding episode of intense activity, a long period of sitting in an awkward position, or a minor muscle strain, but most often there is no causative mechanism. Occasionally, an upper respiratory infection may precede the symptoms and may be implicated as a possible cause. One theory suggests that wry neck is caused by an abnormality of the facet joints opposite the side to which the head is flexed.

Physical examination shows pain in the neck with possible palpable muscle spasm; range of motion is usually limited by the pain. The neurologic examination yields no abnormal findings. Differential diagnosis includes muscular strain, cervical disk abnormality, and cervical spinal abnormality.

The initial treatment consists of muscle relaxants, analgesics, and local applications of heat. Mobilization of the facet joints may be attempted by using general oscillatory movements with traction; however, if this therapy makes the pain worse, it should be discontinued. If none of the above treatment options is successful, further workup is necessary to rule out abnormalities such as fracture or dislocations.

Criteria for return to play are minimal or no neck tenderness, full active range of motion, normal neck strength, and no signs or symptoms of abnormal neurologic function.

Anterior Neck Trauma

Injuries to the anterior neck can occur in a number of sports, especially hockey, soccer, wrestling, and martial arts. Injuries can occur to the trachea, the larynx, and the hyoid bone, and may cause serious airway compromise, delayed hemorrhage, or laryngospasm. If these injuries are suspected, the ABCDs of resuscitative care should be used immediately as needed. Equipment for an emergency airway must be readily available. Return to play depends on the severity of the injury.

Contusion

Direct trauma to the cervical area from an elbow, hand, knee, foot, or even athletic equipment can cause a contusion. Contusion can be a muscle, bone, or nerve injury. The pain usually is localized, and range of motion is limited. Physical examination may show localized tenderness, swelling, ecchymosis, and restricted range of motion, and possibly pain with forward flexion (fractured spinous process) or weakness of shoulder musculature (injury to a nerve). Treatment depends on the anatomic structures involved; that is, it is related to the specific location of the contusion. If the contusion is muscular, ice, protection, stretching, and strengthening are indicated. If fracture is suspected, orthopedic referral is necessary. If the contusion is neural, all motor or sensory deficits should be resolved and strength should be normal before the athlete is allowed to return to competition.

Cervical Strain

Cervical strain is an injury to the muscle–tendon unit caused by overloading or excessive stretching. The muscles most commonly involved are the trapezius, the sternocleidomastoid, the erector spinae, the scalenus, the levator scapulae, and the rhomboids. Mechanisms of injury include hyperextension, hyperflexion, rotation, and ipsilateral side bending. Pain occurring at the time of injury may subside after a few minutes. However, as blood accumulates in the torn muscle fibers, pain, swelling, and tenderness develop, and range of motion is usually limited. Symptoms may not peak until after several hours, or even the next day. Differential diagnosis includes acute torticollis, cervical disk lesions, cervical spine injury, and complete muscle rupture.

The initial treatment includes ice, rest, and anti-inflammatory agents. Heat, massage, ultrasound, and other therapeutic modalities may be added as needed. Once the pain has subsided a gentle stretching and strengthening program should be instituted. The criteria for return to play relevant to the previously discussed injuries apply to this injury as well.

Cervical Sprain

A cervical sprain is an injury to the ligamentous and capsular structures connecting the facet joints and the vertebrae. The injury may result from a compression, wherein the athlete complains of having "jammed" his or her neck, from hyperextension, or from hyperflexion.

There is usually neck pain, and range of motion is limited. Initially, there is no radiation of pain or paresthesia; however, the pain may soon radiate along the muscle groups overlying the area of injury. The neurologic findings are usually normal, although there may be associated neurologic involvement if extensive ligamentous disruption has occurred and instability of the vertebrae is present. The differential diagnosis includes cervical strain, acute torticollis, and cervical fracture.

The cervical spine should be examined by radiographic studies. A complete cervical series with neck flexion and extension views to rule out fracture and dislocation and to document stability is necessary when bone injury is suspected. Magnetic resonance imaging should be reserved for those injuries in which cervical cord contusion or ligamentous instability is possible.

Treatment for sprains without instability or neurologic findings includes brief immobilization, anti-inflammatory or analgesic medications, and application of ice. Once pain has subsided an active rehabilitation program with strengthening is helpful. If the patient has severe pain and muscle spasm, hospitalization with halter traction or a halo brace may be necessary.

The risk of reinjury is high, and chronic inflammatory changes can occur if the athlete returns to competition before complete healing has occurred. Criteria for return to play are full, pain-free range of motion, no paresthesias, and complete return of muscle strength.

Cervical Spinal Cord Neuropraxia with Transient Quadriplegia

The spinal cord is normally well protected by the spinal canal of the cervical vertebrae. Certain conditions, however, can predispose an athlete to spinal cord injury. The athlete with obvious cervical spinal stenosis, congenital fusions, cervical instability, or intervertebral disk protrusions associated with a decrease in the anteroposterior diameter of the spinal canal is at risk of cervical spinal cord neuropraxia with transient quadriplegia. The injury can be caused by forced hyperextension, hyperflexion, or axial loading to the cervical spine in the at-risk athlete. Mechanical compression of the cord results in symptoms in at least two extremities: burning pain, numbness, tingling or loss of sensation, weakness, or complete paralysis. The episodes are transient, with complete recovery usually occurring in 10 to 15 minutes, although an occasional episode may last for 36 to 48 hours. Neck pain is not present at the time of injury, and there is complete return of motor function and full, pain-free cervical motion. A complete and detailed neurologic examination should be carried out, and x-rays of the cervical spine should be obtained. Magnetic resonance imaging (MRI) scans need not be obtained routinely.

Cervical spinal stenosis in an asymptomatic athlete does not predispose the athlete to permanent neurologic injury. The risk of recurring neuropraxia among symptomatic football players with cervical stenosis who have returned to play has been reported to be 50%. The return of such an athlete to contact sports must be evaluated on an individual basis. Absolute contraindications to continued participation after a documented episode of neuropraxia are (1) ligamentous instability, (2) intervertebral disk disease, (3) degenerative changes, (4) MRI scan evidence of defects, swelling, or spinal stenosis, (5)

resolved. Careful, repeated neurologic examinations are necessary to follow the progression and resolution of deficits. X-rays, electromyograms, and MRI scans should be obtained as needed on a case-by-case basis.

Rehabilitation for brachial plexus injuries should include not only a complete shoulder-strengthening program, but also a strengthening program for the trapezius, the latissimus dorsi, the chest musculature, and the musculature distal to the shoulder. Return to play should be deferred until these programs are completed.

Rehabilitation

Rehabilitation for neck injuries not only is important in treatment but also can prevent future injuries. Rehabilitation should be injury-specific, but two basic principles apply: range of motion and muscular strength. Range-of-motion exercises include those movements that are assessed in the physical examination. They include neck flexion, neck extension, lateral bending, and lateral rotation. This specific exercise should be done either in the sitting or the standing position. The exercises are done for 10 to 15 seconds, followed by relaxation, and are repeated 6 to 10 times.

Strength

Once range of motion has been established, regaining muscle strength is important for the athlete to return to competition. Although the protocol should be injury-specific, basic strengthening programs will be discussed. Methods of muscle strengthening for the neck fall under two main categories: isometric and isotonic (see Chapter 5 for further information).

Similar to the rehabilitation of extremity injuries, strength training following a neck injury is usually started with isometric exercise. The athlete is asked to perform sets of repetitive contractions against a nonmoving resistance. This can be easily done by using the athlete's hand as a counterforce. The athlete pushes the head with the hand and resists this motion with a contraction of the neck muscles. Both flexion-extension and side bending can be strengthening in this isometric fashion.

Once the strength improves without further neck pain, isotonic exercise can be done with elastic tubing or special weight equipment that attaches to the head. This time actual flexion-extension and side-bending movement is accomplished against resistance. In athletes with chronic neck injuries this is not always well tolerated, and isometric exercise may be the only choice of strengthening in those cases.

Differential Diagnosis of Neck Pain

Acute Pain

✗ Cervical spine fracture
✗ Cervical spine dislocation
✗ Cervical sprain or strain
✗ Acute torticollis

Chronic Pain

✗ Cervical disk herniation
✗ Degenerative disk disease
✗ Inadequate rehabilitation following acute sprain or strain
✗ Chronic instability following an acute injury

Suggested Readings

Markey KL, Di Benedetto M, Curl WW. The stinger syndrome: upper trunk brachial plexopathy. Am J Sports Med 1993;21:650–655.

McKeag DB, Hough DO. Primary care sports medicine. Dubuque, IA: Brown & Benchmark, 1993.

Nicholas JA, Hershman EB. The upper extremity in sports medicine. St. Louis: CV Mosby, 1990.

Reid DC. Injuries and conditions of the neck and spine. In: Sports injury assessment and rehabilitation. New York: Churchill Livingstone, 1992;739–837.

Roaf R. A study of the mechanics of spinal injuries. J Bone Joint Surg 1960;42B:810–823.

Torg JS. Athletic injuries to the head, neck, and face. 2nd ed. St. Louis: Mosby Year Book, 1991.

Torg JS, Glasgow SG. Criteria for return to contact activities after cervical spine injury. Clin J Sports Med 1991;1:12–26.

Torg JS, Truex R Jr, Quedenfeld TC, et al. The National Football Head and Neck Injury Registry. Report and conclusions 1978. JAMA 1979;241:1477–1478.

Watkins RG. Neck injuries in football players. Clin Sports Med 1986;5:215–246.

CHAPTER 7

Shoulder Injuries

Louis C. Almekinders

The shoulder joint is one of the most commonly injured joints in athletics. Only knee injuries and in some sports hand injuries are more common than shoulder injuries. The shoulder joint is vulnerable to acute injuries not only from direct impact but also as a result of indirect forces such as a fall on the outstretched arm. In indirect injuries the entire upper extremity can act as a long lever arm, thereby amplifying the forces that are exerted on the shoulder joint. Chronic shoulder injuries are extremely common in sports with heavy use of the upper extremity such as swimming, throwing, and racquet sports.

Besides the large forces that are exerted on the shoulder joint during sports, the anatomic features of the shoulder joint contribute to its vulnerability to injury. The shoulder joint is one of the most mobile in the body. It allows a large range of motion in virtually every plane. In order to allow this mobility, the joint has little intrinsic stability owing to the bony contours of the joint. Most of the stability is provided by the surrounding soft tissues, which include the ligaments and muscle-tendon units. This delicate balance between mobility and soft tissue stability makes the shoulder joint prone to acute and chronic injuries. This chapter will describe in more detail the soft tissue anatomy and injuries around the shoulder joint complex.

Anatomy

The shoulder complex consists of more than one joint. Most of the motion of the shoulder occurs in the joint between the humerus and

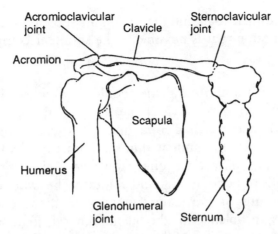

Figure 7.1 *The shoulder complex with the scapula, humerus, and clavicle. Both glenohumeral and acromioclavicular joints are shown.* (Reproduced by permission from Richmond J, Shahady E. Sports medicine for primary care. Cambridge, MA: Blackwell Science, 1995.)

glenoid socket of the scapula, the glenohumeral joint (Fig. 7.1). In a normal glenohumeral joint approximately 120° of forward elevation or flexion is possible. The remaining motion that is possible (with a total of approximately 180°) occurs in the scapulathoracic joint. The shoulder blade or scapula is connected to the chest wall or thorax through muscles. There is also a small joint between the acromion of the scapula and collarbone or clavicle, the acromioclavicular (AC) joint (Fig. 7.2). The movement of muscles between the

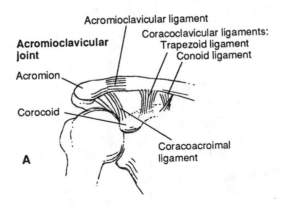

Figure 7.2 *The acromioclavicular joint and its ligaments.* (Reproduced by permission from Richmond J, Shahady E. Sports medicine for primary care. Cambridge, MA: Blackwell Science, 1995.)

scapulathoracic joint and the AC joint contributes significantly to the overall motion that is possible in the shoulder complex.

Ligaments

Ligaments in and around the shoulder complex play an important role in the stability of the joint. In general the ligaments are less defined than those in a joint like the knee. In the shoulder joint they are thickened bands within the joint capsule, rather than separate bands as in the knee joint. However, their integrity is crucial for a normally functioning shoulder joint. The anterior glenohumeral ligaments are of particular importance because the majority of instability problems in the glenohumeral joint involve anterior instability. Superior, middle, and inferior anterior glenohumeral ligaments have been identified (Fig. 7.3). The posterior glenohumeral ligaments are less clearly defined. The stability of the AC joint is provided by both acromioclavicular and coracoclavicular ligaments (see Fig. 7.2).

Muscle-Tendon Units

Significant muscle power is needed to move a mobile joint like the shoulder and provide a stable platform for the rest of the upper extremity to work on. In addition to the ligamentous structures, the muscle-tendon units provide stability to the shoulder joint. Numerous muscles stabilize and move the scapulothoracic joint. Some of the important scapular stabilizers are the rhomboids, levator scapulae, serratus anterior, and the trapezius muscles (Fig. 7.4). The rhomboids

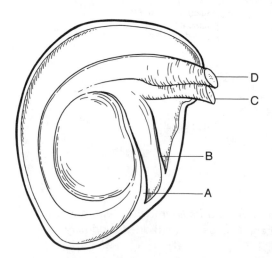

Figure 7.3 *Inside view of the glenoid socket with the anterior glenohumeral ligaments (inferior A, middle B, and superior C) and biceps tendon (D).*

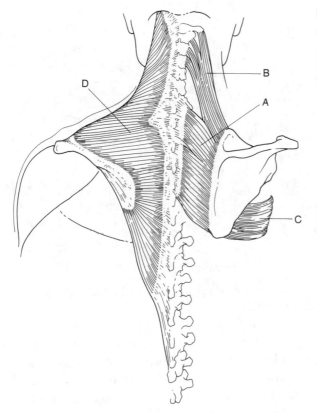

Figure 7.4 *The periscapular muscles including rhomboids (A), levator scapulae (B), serratus anterior (C), and trapezius (D).*

primarily serve to retract the scapula toward the midline. The serratus anterior keeps the scapula stabilized against the thorax during forceful upper extremity activities. Loss of serratus power therefore results in winging of the scapula. The trapezius and levator are capable of pulling the scapula superiorly.

The muscles that surround the glenohumeral joint also have the dual role of stabilization and motion. The deepest layer of muscles is the rotator cuff. It consists of four muscles: the subscapularis in the front, the supraspinatus superiorly, and the infraspinatus and teres minor in the back (Fig. 7.5). In this way they surround the glenohumeral joint approximately 270°. This group of muscles primarily functions to keep the humeral head well seated in the glenoid socket. In addition, the supraspinatus provides abduction; the subscapularis, internal rotation; and the infraspinatus and teres minor, external rotation power.

Superficial to the rotator cuff lies the deltoid muscle. It is divided in anterior middle, and posterior segments that provide internal rota-

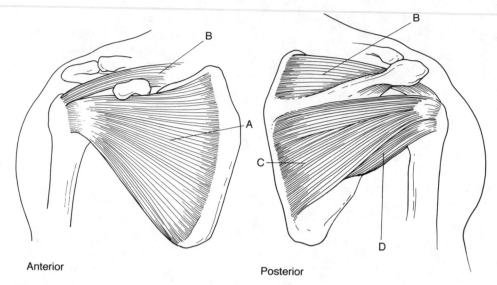

Anterior

Posterior

Figure 7.5 *The rotator cuff muscles consist of subscapularis (A), supraspinatus (B), infraspinatus (C), and teres minor (D).*

tion, abduction, and external rotation power, respectively. Other muscles that cross the shoulder joint are the biceps, pectoralis major, and latissimus dorsi. The latter two provide adduction and additional rotatory power to the shoulder. The biceps had a long and a short head. The long head passes between the subscapularis and supraspinatus insertion in the humerus and enters the glenohumeral joint. It attaches to the superior rim of the glenoid socket and thereby acts as another stabilizer of the glenohumeral joint.

Cartilage

The glenohumeral joint is covered by articular cartilage as is found in any synovial joint. In addition to this articular cartilage, a special fibrocartilaginous structure can be found in this joint, somewhat analogous to the meniscus in the knee joint. The shoulder joint capsule attaches to the edge of the glenoid. This edge is a fibrocartilaginous rim called the labrum (Fig. 7.6). In addition to serving as a capsular attachment point, it deepens the otherwise superficial glenoid and thereby provides further stability to the shoulder joint.

Bursa

Several bursae have been described around the shoulder. Of particular importance is the subdeltoid or subacromial bursa. This bursa is located directly superficial to the rotator cuff but deep to the deltoid

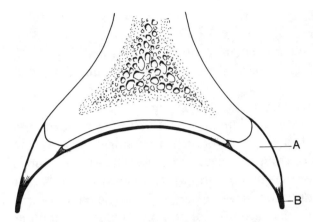

Figure 7.6 *A cross section of the glenoid socket with labrum (A) and capsule (B).*

and the acromion. Its function is to allow smooth motion between the rotator cuff tendons and the acromion.

Acute Shoulder Injuries

Acute soft tissue injuries frequently occur in athletics as the result of a direct force of the shoulder or upper extremity. This section will discuss the most common acute injuries. In addition to intrinsic shoulder injuries, it is possible that acute shoulder pain can be found as referred pain from areas outside the shoulder. Cervical spine problems and cardiac and pulmonary diseases are notorious for their referred pain to the shoulder and upper extremity. Extrinsic causes should be kept in mind when evaluating an athlete with shoulder pain.

Shoulder Dislocation

A complete displacement of the humeral head out of the glenoid socket is termed a shoulder dislocation. A lesser degree of displacement is called a shoulder subluxation. As opposed to the subluxation, dislocation often persists after it has occurred. The humeral head is often trapped outside the rim of the glenoid, and a reduction maneuver is needed to replace the head back into the glenoid. In most subluxations the head slips back into the glenoid spontaneously. The problem of recurrent subluxations will be discussed below in the section on chronic shoulder injuries.

The vast majority of shoulder dislocations involve an anterior displacement of the humeral head relative to the socket. The mechanism of injury is associated with the arm in an abducted, externally rotated, and hyperextended position. In this position the humeral head is levered anteriorly over the edge of the glenoid and becomes trapped under the coracoid process.

The symptoms include immediate severe pain and inability to use the arm. On physical examination the dislocated humeral head is often visible and palpable anteriorly. Occasionally an axillary nerve palsy is present as well owing to traction on the nerve. This will result in decreased sensation over the lateral aspect of the upper arm and weakness of the deltoid. X-rays are obtained to confirm the direction of the dislocation and rule out associated fractures. It is important to always obtain x-rays of the shoulder in two different directions that are 90° opposed to one another (Fig. 7.7). A single view of the shoulder can appear deceivingly normal in some cases of shoulder dislocations.

The initial treatment of a dislocated shoulder is a reduction of the humeral head. Several maneuvers can accomplish this. One relatively gentle method is by placing the patient prone on the edge of the table with the affected arm hanging down. Administration of an analgesic or muscle relaxant or both as well as the application of a weight to the arm can be of help. If this is not successful, other more forceful methods have been described but are beyond the scope of this chapter.

Following the reduction x-rays should be repeated to confirm a complete reduction. The arm is placed in a sling, and ice and analge-

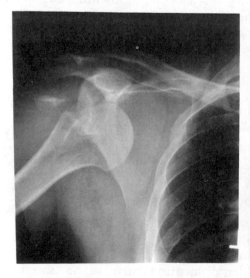 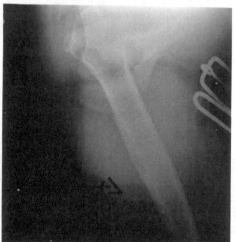

Figure 7.7 *Anteroposterior view (A) and axillary view (B) of a dislocated shoulder.*

sics are used in the first few days. The length of immobilization in a sling is quite controversial. A shoulder dislocation can result in clear damage to the anterior glenohumeral ligaments or the labral and capsular attachments at the anterior rim of the glenoid. A complete labrum detachment is termed a Bankart lesion. However, it has not been proved conclusively that prolonged immobilization significantly affects the healing of these structures. Both with and without prolonged immobilization, incomplete healing of these injured structures is extremely common in young athletes. This leads to shoulder instability with recurrent dislocations often after trivial trauma. Repeat dislocations have been reported in as many as 80% to 90% of patients in their teens and twenties. The risk of recurrent dislocations decreases significantly with increasing age at the time of first dislocation. A sling is used anywhere from 2 to 6 weeks depending on the treating physician's preference.

More important than the length of immobilization is the rehabilitation. After the sling is discontinued gentle range-of-motion exercises are started but extreme external rotation is avoided. External rotation causes particular stretch of the injured structures. This is followed by a vigorous strengthening program with emphasis on the internal rotators such as the anterior deltoid and subscapularis muscles. These muscles are thought to be important in preventing repeat dislocation. Return to full activities will take a minimum of 2 to 3 months depending on the type of sport that is involved.

Shoulder or Acromioclavicular Joint Separation

A shoulder separation is an injury of the ligaments of the AC joint. This can occur with a direct fall onto the tip of the shoulder but also indirectly through a fall onto an outstretched arm. A rupture of the ligaments surrounding the AC joint will allow the shoulder to sag down more than usual. This leads to a separation of the AC joint with a prominent distal end of the clavicle (Fig. 7.8). The injury to the ligaments can vary in severity, and thereby the amount of the separation can vary. Three basic degrees of separation are seen (see Fig. 7.8). Other types of separation are possible but fortunately quite rare.

The symptoms of an AC separation are immediate pain and sometimes a prominence on the top of the shoulder. Unlike a shoulder dislocation, gentle rotation of the arm is not particularly painful because this takes place in the glenohumeral joint, which is not affected.

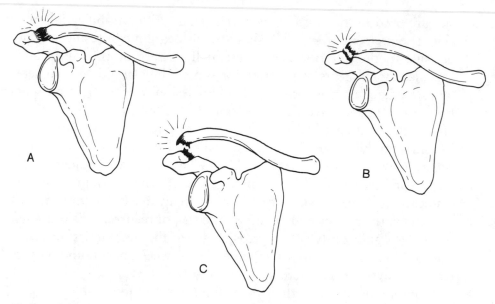

Figure 7.8 *First-degree (A), second-degree (B), and third-degree (C) AC joint separations.*

Initial treatment also includes a sling for comfort, ice, and analgesics. Definitive treatment is somewhat controversial, but most studies report good results with symptomatic treatment only, without any attempt to reduce the separation. Reduction of the separation in most cases would require a surgical procedure with ligament repair and placement of hardware to keep the AC joint reduced. The complications and recovery time associated with this type of surgery are generally thought to be outweighed by the benefits of nonsurgical treatment. Nonsurgical treatment includes range-of-motion and strengthening exercises as soon as the patient's level of pain allows them. Return to sports is often possible in several weeks. The return of both flexibility and strength is generally excellent. The main risk is the development of late AC joint arthritis if the joint is left partially separated. However, a small surgical procedure with removal of the distal end of the clavicle generally solves this problem if it occurs.

Rotator Cuff Tears

Acute tears of a previously healthy rotator cuff are relatively rare. Most tears are the end result of a chronic injury that affected the cuff. The diagnosis and treatment of rotator cuff tears will be discussed below in the section on chronic shoulder injuries.

Biceps Tendon Ruptures

The tendon of the long head of the biceps muscle is susceptible to rupture. This can occur in young athletes with a violent contraction of the biceps and simultaneous stretch due to external forces. In older athletes it may be associated with a degenerative lesion near the origin of the tendon at the superior rim of the glenoid.

The symptoms are a sudden pain and appearance of a bulge near the upper half of the biceps muscle. Treatment is usually symptomatic in older athletes. The loss of strength is usually small owing to the presence of an intact short head of the biceps. In power athletes surgical reconstruction can be considered. Repair is usually not possible, but the ruptured tendon can be attached to the proximal humerus. This preserves some of the biceps power at the elbow.

Fractures

An extensive description of fractures around the shoulder is beyond the scope of this book. However, the possibility of a fracture should be kept in mind when evaluating an injured shoulder. The most common fracture around the shoulder is a clavicle fracture. Although painful, it has an excellent healing rate with symptomatic treatment only. Proximal humerus fractures also occur and can pose a more serious problem. Displaced proximal humerus fractures often require surgical reduction and internal fixation for an optimal result.

Chronic Shoulder Injuries

Chronic shoulder injuries are at least as common as acute injuries. They are particularly common in athletes who swim, throw, or use, racquets, because of the cumulative effect of the repetitive motion that is involved in these activities. The diagnosis of these injuries can be difficult. This is partly due to the considerable overlap between some of the injuries. The knowledge that allows one to evaluate and treat these injuries has only emerged in the past 5 to 10 years. Further research is still needed to fully understand the pathology in some of these injuries.

Impingement Syndrome

The word *syndrome* implies a constellation of signs and symptoms without necessarily knowing the exact cause of the problem. Impingement syndrome in the shoulder indeed reflects a fairly wide variety of signs and symptoms; however, the potential causes of this syndrome are becoming more clear with new research in the past several years. These studies indicate that one of the aspects of this syndrome is the impingement of the soft tissue between the acromion and the humerus. With forward flexion and abduction of the humerus, the space between the acromion and humerus becomes smaller (Fig. 7.9). This space is occupied by the rotator cuff and the subacromial bursa. Normally these soft tissue structures tolerate this occasional impingement quite well. However, if the impingement is extremely repetitive or excessive in nature, an impingement syndrome can develop. In the early stages this results in a combination of subacromial bursitis and rotator cuff tendinitis. If the impingement persists and the tendinitis becomes chronic, the lesion can progress to a rotator cuff tear. As the supraspinatus tendon is particularly prone to impingement, tendinitis and tears are most commonly found in that part of the rotator cuff.

The symptoms of impingement syndrome are dominated by pain. Initially the pain is present mainly in activities that create the impingement. Most activities that require shoulder forward flexion beyond the level of the shoulder bring on the pain. This is particularly disabling for throwing athletes, swimmers, and those involved in

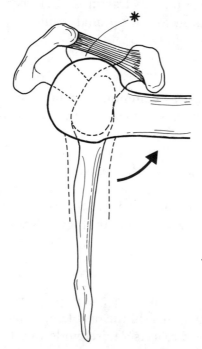

Figure 7.9 *Mechanism of impingement (*) with forward flexion of the humerus.*

racquet sports. If the syndrome progresses, the pain may also be present at rest. Pain at night is a common problem in patients with chronic rotator cuff problems. Many athletes will sense that their arm is weak as well. This may indicate a rotator cuff tear, or the weakness may merely be subjective secondary to the pain with activity.

Physical examination is based on provoking the impingement. Bringing the arm in passive forward flexion will often reproduce the pain at approximately 80° to 90°. Additional internal rotation will often aggravate the pain because it narrows the subacromial space even more. Palpation of the subacromial space may also elicit some of the pain. Many physicians will attempt to place some local anesthetic such as lidocaine into the subacromial space by an injection through the deltoid muscle. An impingement syndrome is quite likely if the majority of the pain with forward flexion disappears following the injection. If a rotator cuff tear is present as well, the diagnostic injection will also improve the pain, but the weakness from the tear will not disappear. If the weakness is only subjective and results from the associated the pain, the injection will also improve the apparent strength. The supraspinatus strength is best tested with the arm in 90° of forward flexion and slight abduction (Fig. 7.10). Both arms are tested simultaneously in order to detect a difference.

Further diagnostic procedures are usually not necessary unless the symptoms are resistant to treatment. The initial treatment is focused on decreasing the irritation caused by the impingement. Relative rest is generally needed and can be accomplished by decreasing the frequency and intensity of the offending motion to a degree that the pain is not felt. For instance, tennis players may have to decrease or stop their serving and overhead swings, swimmers may have to resort to

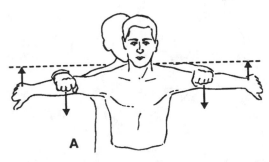

Figure 7.10 *Strength testing of the supraspinatus muscles.* (Reproduced by permission from Richmond J, Shahady E. Sports medicine for primary care. Cambridge, MA: Blackwell Science, 1995.)

swimming with a kickboard only, and throwers may have to decrease the speed and frequency of their pitching. In addition, nonsteroidal anti-inflammatory drugs and icing can be of help in decreasing the pain. Once the initial pain has subsided, rehabilitative exercises become extremely important. Stretching the rotator cuff muscles can correct tightness in other parts of the cuff and stimulate a healing response. Subsequently rotator cuff strengthening exercises can also stimulate the healing. In addition, the pain often has caused secondary cuff weakness and dysfunction, which worsens the impingement itself as the weak cuff is unable to contain the humeral head in the glenoid socket. Of similar importance is strengthening of the scapular-stabilizing muscles. Poor posture and chronic pain can cause a forward rotation of the scapula. This allows the acromion to turn down more, and impingement occurs with fewer degrees of forward flexion (Fig. 7.11).

If in 6 to 12 weeks there has been no or minimal response to the initial treatment, further investigations may be helpful. X-rays of the shoulder can allow one to rule out other problems such as glenohumeral arthritis. In addition, they can give information regard-

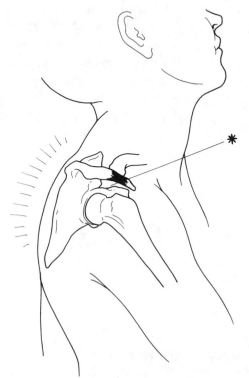

Figure 7.11 *Poor posture with increased chance of impingement (*) due to scapular positioning.*

ing the shape of the acromion. If this shape is relatively curved or hooked, it is more likely that impingement is the primary problem and surgical treatment may be beneficial. Before resorting to surgical treatment a steroid injection into the subacromial space is often attempted. The corticosteroids are strong anti-inflammatory drugs but also weaken collagenous tissues like those of the rotator cuff. Therefore it is recommended to temporarily decrease shoulder exercise following a steroid injection. Normal activities are often gradually restarted after 2 to 3 weeks of relative rest. If the pain persists and no rotator cuff tear is present, the impingement syndrome can be treated surgically. An arthroscopic subacromial decompression will remove some of the bone at the undersurface of the acromion, thereby allowing more room for the cuff and the bursa and decreasing the impingement.

If the pain remains resistant and objective weakness is also a problem, a rotator cuff tear may be present. Many rotator cuff tears are thought to represent an end stage of chronic cuff tendinitis. This is complicated by the fact that the supraspinatus has a poor blood supply and seems susceptible to degeneration even without an overt impingement syndrome. Once a tear occurs, little or no spontaneous healing seems to occur. Although most patients assume an acute increase in their pain as the time of onset, it seems likely that the tearing is actually a chronic process.

If supraspinatus weakness and atrophy is noted, a tear should be suspected. Arthrography, magnetic resonance imaging (MRI) scan (Fig. 7.12), or arthroscopy can objectively determine the presence of such tears. If present in young athletes, they are generally surgically repaired to avoid chronic weakness.

Secondary Impingement Syndrome

Not every athlete with signs and symptoms of impingement has a pure impingement syndrome. In some cases the impingement is secondary to another problem in the shoulder. The most common problem resulting in secondary impingement is shoulder subluxation. When this is present, the underlying subluxation should be primarily treated and not only the impingement. Recurrent subluxation will be discussed in the following section.

Recurrent Anterior Subluxation

Normally the glenoid labrum and the glenohumeral ligaments are the static restraints that prevent subluxation or dislocation of the hu-

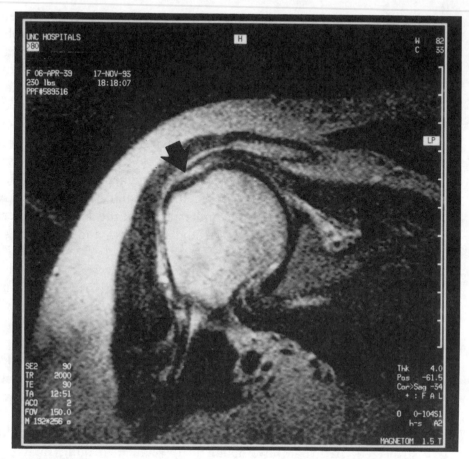

Figure 7.12 *MRI scan of a shoulder with a rotator cuff tear (arrow).*

meral head out of the glenoid socket. These structures can become insufficient through acute or chronic injury. The acute injury most commonly responsible for this is a shoulder dislocation as discussed in the section above on acute shoulder injuries. Chronically, the injury can occur due to repetitive stresses placed on these structures. Again, the overhead throwing motion is largely responsible for this. During the throwing motion the arm is often placed in extreme abduction and external rotation. This places a large stress on the anterior glenohumeral ligaments and the labrum, which can lead to gradual stretching of the ligament and tearing of the glenoid labrum. Once the ligaments and labrum have become insufficient through chronic or acute injury, the humeral head will tend to subluxate anteriorly every time the arm is placed in abduction and external rotation.

The symptoms of recurrent subluxation often involve acute episodes of shoulder pain, particularly when the arm is placed in abduction and external rotation. The athlete will quickly drop the arm and often describe this as a "dead arm." Between the episodes of subluxation the shoulder is often relatively asymptomatic unless there is an element of secondary impingement (see previous section).

On clinical examination this recurrent anterior subluxation can be brought out by provoking the "apprehension sign." The arm is placed in 90° of abduction and maximal external rotation. The examiner then places one hand on the humeral head posteriorly and holds the patient's wrist with the other (Fig. 7.13). Additional pressure on the humeral head combined with forced external rotation through the wrist will caused marked pain and apprehension in the athlete with an unstable shoulder. Occasionally there will also be a positive impingement test as a result of secondary impingement caused by the instability (see previous section).

The initial treatment of recurrent anterior subluxation can involve a decrease in those activities that provoke the subluxation. Stretching, particularly of the posterior rotator cuff, is started. In throwing athletes this part of the cuff is often tight. Posterior cuff force adds to the problem of subluxation as the tight muscle pushes the humeral head anteriorly into the deficient side of the joint. In addition, rotator cuff strengthening exercises with an emphasis on the subscapularis muscle are started. Because the subscapularis overlies the anterior shoulder capsule, it is thought that strengthening this muscle can

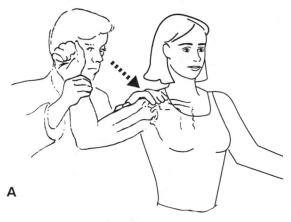

A

Figure 7.13 *Apprehension test for shoulder subluxation.* (Reproduced by permission from Richmond J, Shahady E. Sports medicine for primary care. Cambridge, MA: Blackwell Science, 1995.)

compensate for insufficient anterior glenohumeral ligaments. If after 3 to 4 months the strengthening is not successful in decreasing the symptoms of subluxation, surgical treatment can be considered. Surgical reconstruction usually involves tightening or repair of the static restraints of the anterior shoulder joint: the anterior glenohumeral ligaments, anterior joint capsule, and anterior labrum. Often this can be done arthroscopically. However, it should be remembered that this type of reconstructive surgery often improves the mechanics of the joint but rarely returns it to normal. A perfect balance between stability and mobility is difficult to obtain with surgery. Elite throwing athletes can often not regain their preinjury competitive level after surgery despite an improvement in their stability.

In persons with secondary impingement a surgical arthroscopic decompression alone should be avoided. Although this is often helpful in cases of primary impingement, it does not address the essential pathology in secondary impingement.

Multidirectional Instability

Some athletes with symptoms of anterior shoulder subluxation also have symptoms and findings suggestive of additional pathology. Feelings of subluxation occur not only in the abducted and externally rotated position but also with neutral abduction and extension. Traction on the arm can reveal a sulcus sign indicative of inferior subluxation (Fig. 7.14). This also indicates that the shoulder joint is

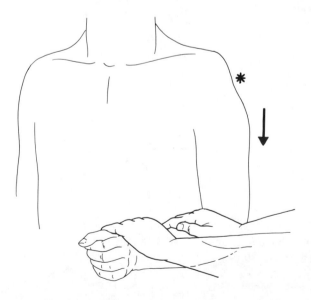

Figure 7.14 *Sulcus sign (*) due to inferior subluxation.*

unstable in more than one direction. Combined anterior and inferior instability is not uncommon. This can occur after an injury but is also seen in congenitally lax individuals without any precipitating injury. Treatment can be very difficult, and surgery is often attempted to control the symptoms. An open reconstructive procedure is generally needed to tighten the joint in several directions.

Arthritis

Degenerative arthritis of the glenohumeral joint is fortunately rare. Even in patients with a history of multiple dislocations, arthritis is still not common. Presumably, this is because the glenohumeral joint is a large but non-weight-bearing joint.

On the other hand, degenerative arthritis of the acromioclavicular joint is not uncommon. The usual cause is a previous AC joint separation in athletes. The minor grades of this injury leave the AC joint chronically subluxed. This can lead to degenerative arthritis, usually within several years.

The symptoms include pain in the area of the AC joint with vigorous activities with the shoulder in forward flexion and abduction. Common examples are bench pressing and pass protection by football linemen.

Treatment includes a decrease in activities and oral anti-inflammatory medication. If this is not successful, an intra-articular steroid injection can be attempted. The relief obtained by these measures is often temporary. Definitive treatment is surgical removal of the outer part of the clavicle. This completely removes the painful, subluxed joint and allows the area to be filled in with scar tissue.

Frozen Shoulder

As opposed to instability in younger athletes, the glenohumeral joint is particularly prone to stiffening in older athletes. This generally does not occur as an isolated problem. The frozen shoulder or adhesive capsulitis is often precipitated by another pain in or around the shoulder that resulted in prolonged immobilization. Typical examples are fractures or dislocations that were immobilized in a sling for several weeks in older patients. Whenever possible motion exercises should be started early after an injury to avoid these problems.

Once a frozen shoulder has developed abduction, forward flexion, and external rotation are often markedly restricted. Physical therapy with an emphasis on stretching exercises is often used to regain this motion. In spite of intense therapy, a frozen shoulder can be chronic and take many months to resolve.

Shoulder Rehabilitation

Rehabilitation following shoulder injuries is extremely important for several reasons. First, the key to improving the symptoms often involves stretching tight structures and strengthening those that are weak. Second, the injury can lead to quick stiffening and weakening, which should be avoided to allow early return to normal activities. Finally, future or recurrent injury can be prevented through adequate rehabilitation. This section will review some of the basic stretching and strengthening exercises often used in shoulder rehabilitation.

Stretching Exercises

Stretching the soft tissues around the glenohumeral complex consists of three basic exercises (Fig. 7.15). The other arm is used as an active assist in these exercises. The posterior cuff and capsular structures are stretched by placing the arm in a forward flexed and adducted position. The anterior structures are stretched by placing the arm behind the back in an abducted and extended position. The inferior capsule is stretched by fully abducting the arm behind the head. These stretches are performed slowly and held for 3 to 4 seconds each time. A set of stretches often includes 5 to 10 stretches before going on to the next set.

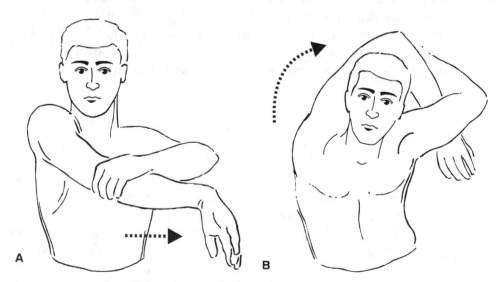

Figure 7.15 *Basic rotator cuff stretching exercises.* (Reproduced by permission from Richmond J, Shahady E. Sports medicine for primary care. Cambridge, MA: Blackwell Science, 1995.)

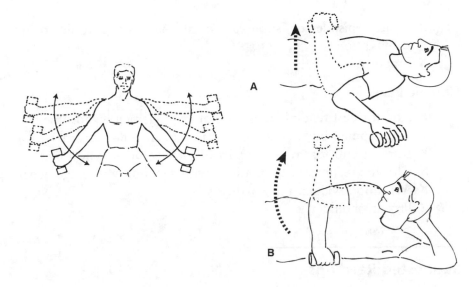

Figure 7.16 *Basic rotator cuff and deltoid strengthening exercises.*
(Reproduced by permission from Richmond J, Shahady E. Sports medicine for
primary care. Cambridge, MA: Blackwell Science, 1995.)

As indicated in the section above on impingement syndrome, not
only the muscles around the glenohumeral joint but also those of
the scapulothoracic joint should be included in the rehabilitation.
This can be accomplished by a variety of exercises. Squeezing the
shoulder blades together is a relatively easy exercise for scapular
retractors. Shoulder shrugging exercises the trapezius and levator
scapulae.

Rotator cuff and deltoid strengthening is often done with free
weights. Three sets of easy cuff and deltoid exercises are shown in
Figure 7.16. Internal and external rotation exercises strengthen the
anterior and posterior cuff and the deltoid muscle, respectively.
Elevation in the scapular plane focuses on the middle deltoid and
supraspinatus muscle.

Differential Diagnosis of Shoulder Pain

Acute Pain

- ✗ Acromioclavicular joint separation
- ✗ Shoulder dislocation

✗ Acute episode of subluxation as part of chronic recurrent subluxation
✗ Fracture

Chronic Pain

✗ Rotator cuff tendinitis (as part of impingement syndrome)
✗ Subacromial bursitis (as part of impingement syndrome)
✗ Rotator cuff tear (may be part of impingement syndrome)
✗ Chronic recurrent subluxation (with secondary impingement)
✗ Acromioclavicular joint arthritis
✗ Frozen shoulder

Suggested Readings

Ellman H, Gartsman GM. Arthroscopic shoulder surgery and related procedures. Malvern, PA: Lea & Febiger, 1993.
Neer CS. Shoulder reconstruction. Philadelphia: WB Saunders, 1990.
Post M, Morrey BF, Hawkins RJ, eds. Surgery of the shoulder. St. Louis: Mosby Year Book, 1990.
Rockwood CA, Matsen FA, eds. The shoulder. Philadelphia: WB Saunders, 1990.

CHAPTER **8**

Elbow Injuries

Charles J. Gatt and Richard D. Parker

The primary function of the elbow is to position the hand in space. Both daily activities and athletic activities require a wide range of elbow flexion, extension, and rotation. Although the elbow is one of the most stable joints in the body, injury due to high-energy and low-energy trauma is not uncommon. The repetitive functional demands of the elbow in athletics also lead to numerous muscle, tendon, ligament, and osseous overuse injuries.

Anatomy

Osseous Anatomy

The elbow joint consists of three articulations between three bones (Fig. 8.1). The distal humerus articulates with the proximal ulna to form the ulnohumeral joint. At this articulation, the trochlea of the distal humerus fits securely into the greater sigmoid notch of the proximal ulna creating a hinge or ginglymus joint. The proximal radius, referred to as the radial head, articulates with the capitellum of the distal humerus creating the radiohumeral or radiocapitellar joint. Slightly distal to the greater sigmoid notch of the ulna, the radial head and ulna articulate to form the proximal radioulnar joint. The radiocapitellar joint and the proximal radioulnar joint allow axial rotation, or trochoid motion, of the forearm and hand. Thus the elbow is classified as a trochoginglymoid joint.

147

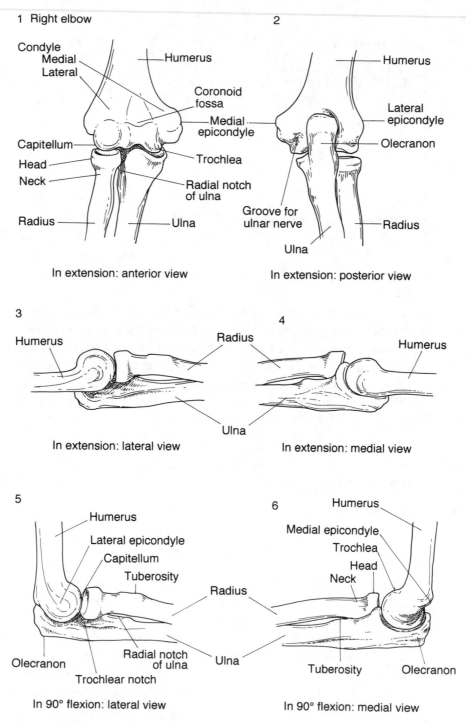

Figure 8.1 *Osseous anatomy.*

Ligamentous Anatomy

The hinged articulation of the ulnohumeral joint provides significant stability to the elbow in the anterior-posterior direction. However, stability of the elbow to varus and valgus rotation is provided primarily by the ligamentous structures. The prime stabilizer of the elbow to valgus rotation is the medial collateral ligament (Fig. 8.2A). The medial collateral ligament consists of three bands, the anterior oblique, the posterior oblique, and the transverse bands. The origin of the medial collateral ligament is on the medial epicondyle of the distal humerus, and it inserts on the medial surface of the proximal ulna. The anterior band is taut with extension, while the posterior band is taut with flexion. The anterior band is the strongest of the three and considered the most significant stabilizer to valgus rotation. The radiocapitellar joint also provides the elbow with stability to

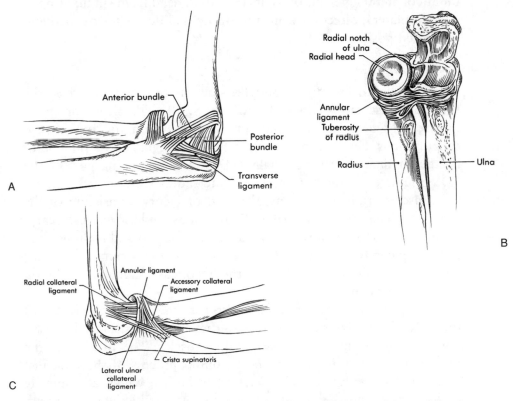

Figure 8.2 *Ligamentous anatomy: medial collateral ligament (A); annular ligament (B); and lateral collateral ligament (C).* (Reproduced by permission from Anderson TE. Anatomy and physical examination of the elbow. In: Nicholas YA, Harshmann EB, eds. The upper extremity in sports medicine. St. Louis: Mosby Year Book, 1990:282–283.)

valgus rotation, however, only after the medial collateral ligament is torn.

On the lateral side of the elbow, the lateral collateral ligament also consists of several components. The annular ligament (Fig. 8.2B) originates anterior to the radial notch of the ulna, wraps around the neck of the radius just distal to the radial head, and inserts posterior to the radial notch of the ulna. Thus it stabilizes the radial head against the ulna while allowing axial rotation of the radius. The radial collateral ligament (Fig. 8.2C) originates on the lateral epicondyle and inserts into the annular ligament. The lateral ulnar collateral ligament (see Fig. 8.2C) originates on the lateral epicondyle and inserts on the lateral surface of the proximal ulna. The lateral collateral ligament serves as a stabilizer to varus rotation. However, its role is not as significant as the medial collateral ligament's. In addition, the lateral ulnar collateral ligament prevents the radial head from subluxating in a posterolateral direction while the elbow is close to an extended and supinated position.

Muscular Anatomy

The medial and lateral epicondyles serve as origins to most of the forearm musculature (Figs. 8.3A and 8.3B). The flexor-pronator muscles originate medially and consist of the pronator teres, flexor carpi radialis, flexor carpi ulnaris, palmaris longus, and a portion of the flexor digitorum superficialis (FDS). The remaining part of the FDS originates on the proximal ulna and radius. Laterally, the extensor muscles originate. The mobile wad of Henry, consisting of the brachioradialis, extensor carpi radialis longus, and the extensor carpi radialis brevis, originates from an area proximal to and including the lateral epicondyle. In addition, the extensor digitorum comminus, part of the supinator muscle, and the anconeus originate distally on the lateral epicondyle.

Posteriorly, the triceps tendon inserts into the olecranon process of the ulna. The anterior musculature of the elbow consists of the distal segments of the biceps and brachialis muscles. The brachialis, the deeper of the two, inserts on the coronoid process of the ulna just distal to the greater sigmoid notch. The biceps, which is primarily tendinous as it crosses the elbow, inserts into the bicipital tuberosity of the proximal radius.

Neurovascular Anatomy

All three of the nerves that innervate the forearm and hand musculature cross the elbow. Posteriorly, the ulnar nerve runs in a groove

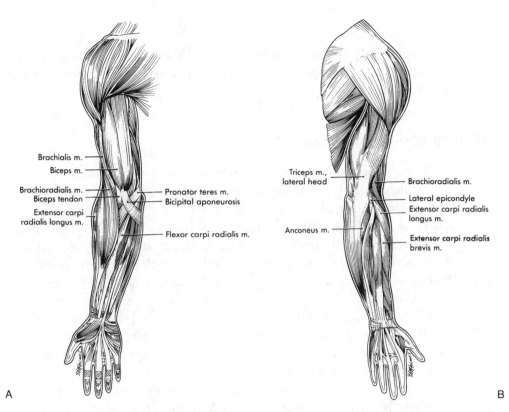

Figure 8.3 *Muscular anatomy: anterior view of the arm (A) and posterior view of the arm (B).* (Reproduced by permission from Anderson TE. Anatomy and physical examination of the elbow. In: Nicholas YA, Harshmann EB, eds. The upper extremity in sports medicine. St. Louis: Mosby Year Book, 1990:282–283.)

behind the medial epicondyle. It courses through the flexor carpi ulnaris, providing innervation, and then onto the forearm and hand. Anterior and lateral, the radial nerve crosses the elbow in the interval between the brachialis and the brachioradialis. Shortly after crossing the elbow, the radial nerve divides into the posterior interosseous nerve, a motor branch, and the superficial radial sensory nerve. Anterior and medial, the median nerve crosses the elbow medial to the biceps tendon. It courses deep to the pronator teres into the forearm and then the hand. The median nerve sends off a motor branch referred to as the anterior interosseous nerve just after it passes the elbow.

The brachial artery and vein run adjacent to the median nerve as it crosses the elbow. At the level of the biceps insertion, the brachial artery divides into the radial and ulnar arteries, which continue into the forearm and hand.

Bursae

Although there are many bursae around the elbow, the olecranon bursa is the one that presents as a clinical entity. It is located on the posterior superficial border of ulna.

History and Physical Examination

Before physical examination of the elbow, a thorough history should be obtained. This provides important information regarding the location of the symptoms, mechanism of injury, and chronicity versus acuteness of the complaint. Initially, establish the chief complaint and whether the injury is acute or chronic. In acute injuries, a description of the activity and the mechanism of injury, such as a direct blow to the elbow or a fall onto an outstretched hand, is necessary information. Ask if the athlete was able to continue participation after the injury or if pain, swelling, or deformity required cessation of the activity. Inquire about the location of maximum pain and maneuvers that increase or decrease discomfort. A history of previous injury to the extremity is also important.

In the patient with a chronic elbow injury, determine the time of onset and duration of symptoms. Ask if the symptoms have worsened, improved, or remained stable over time. Question the athlete regarding sports and daily activities that lead to increased discomfort and if the pain prevents participation in sports or work-related activities. Obtain information concerning previous treatment such as medication, injections, or physical therapy. The information gained by a thorough history will be of considerable help during the physical examination.

The initial part of the physical examination should be inspection of the injured elbow and comparison with the uninvolved elbow. This will aid in the detection of lacerations, swelling, defects, atrophy, hypertrophy, or asymmetry. In addition, a comparison of carrying angles can be made (Figs. 8.4A and 8.4B). The normal elbow in the extended position has a valgus angle of 5° in men and 10° to 15° in women.

Next, active range of motion is tested (Fig. 8.5). Full extension of the elbow is when the forearm and upper arm form a straight line and is recorded as 0°. Most men are able to extend to 0°. Many women can actually extend the elbow to 5° past 0° of extension. This is recorded as −5°. Full flexion of the elbow, approximately 150°,

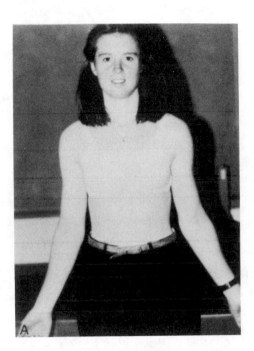
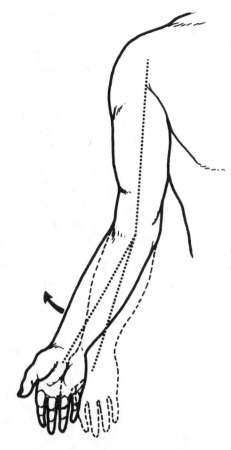

Figure 8.4 *Carrying angle of the elbow.* (Reproduced by permission from Manual of orthopaedic surgery. Chicago: American Orthopaedic Association, 1972:138.)

should allow the patient to touch the shoulder with the hand. Pronation and supination should be measured with the elbow flexed to approximately 90°. The total arc or rotation should be 180°. The zero position is when the hand is parallel to the sagittal plane. Pronation of 90° is obtained when the palm of the hand is facing the floor. Supination of 90° is achieved when the palm is facing directly upward and parallel with the horizontal plane.

Comfortable performance of daily activities requires a flexion-extension arc of 30° to 130° and a pronation-supination arc of 50° of pronation to 50° of supination. Loss of range of motion can be due to soft tissue swelling or scarring, muscle injury or tightness, heterotopic ossification, or intra-articular cartilage damage, loose bodies, or degenerative arthritis.

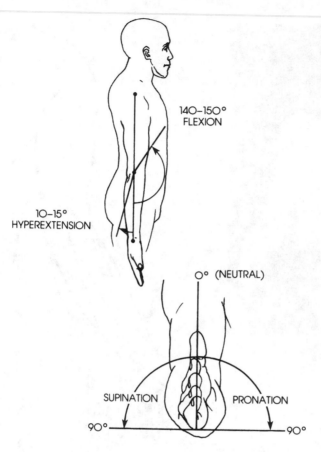

Figure 8.5 *Range of motion of the elbow.* (Reproduced by permission from Magee. Orthopedic physical assessment. Philadelphia: WB Saunders, 1990:147.)

The superficial nature of most bony landmarks in the elbow makes palpation relatively easy. The medial epicondyle, lateral epicondyle, and olecranon process are easily palpable assuming soft tissue swelling is not severe. These three landmarks should form a straight line at 0° of extension and an isosceles triangle with the tip of the olecranon as the apex at 90° of elbow flexion (Fig. 8.6). On the posterior aspect of the medial epicondyle is a groove for the ulnar nerve. Within this groove one can palpate the ulnar nerve as it courses around the posterior aspect of the elbow. The radial head is palpable distal to the lateral epicondyle. Pronation and supination of the forearm with palpation on the lateral elbow will aid in locating the radial head.

The flexor pronator and common extensor muscle origins and muscle bellies are readily palpated on the medial and lateral aspects of the elbow, respectively. Isometric and isotonic contractions of the muscle groups will aid in the location, examination, and strength

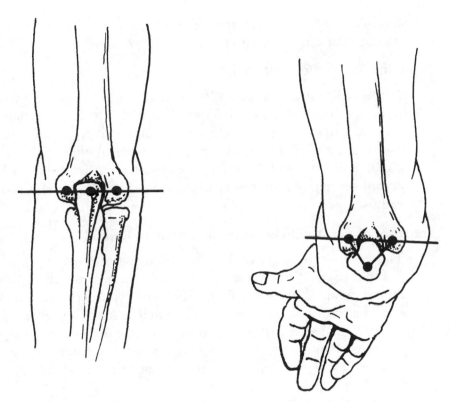

Figure 8.6 *Palpable landmarks of the elbow.* (Reproduced by permission from Magee. Orthopedic physical assessment. Philadelphia: WB Saunders, 1992:147.)

assessment. The triceps musculotendinous junction and the insertion are easily examined in the posterior elbow. Anteriorly, the biceps tendon can be palpated, and isometric contraction again aids in location. Medial to the biceps tendon, the pulse of the brachial artery is detectable.

An enlarged or inflamed olecranon bursa can be palpated along the superficial border of the proximal ulna. Also, supracondylar lymph nodes are palpable on the posteromedial aspect of the elbow.

Acute Injuries of the Elbow

Acute injuries of the elbow generally result from an indirect load on the elbow. Athletes invariably attempt to dampen the impact of a fall by bracing themselves with one or both outstretched arms. If the impact is too great, injuries can occur at wrist, elbow, or shoulder level. The most common acute elbow injuries in children and adults are discussed in this section.

Acute Injuries of the Pediatric Elbow

In the skeletally immature athlete, osseous injuries are more common than ligament and tendon injuries. This is due to the presence of the physeal growth plates of the distal humerus, proximal ulna, and radius and the relative weakness of metaphyseal bone in the growing child. Fractures will be briefly discussed in order to describe the complete range of injuries possible around the elbow and proximal radius.

Fractures of the Distal Humerus and Proximal Radius

The most severe injury of the elbow in this group is a supracondylar fracture of the distal humerus. The mechanism is usually a fall onto an outstretched arm (Fig. 8.7). This injury is associated with severe swelling, neuropraxic injuries to the radial or median nerves, vascular injuries, and compartment syndromes of the forearm. Displaced fractures require prompt surgical treatment. Minimally displaced fractures will not manifest as dramatically and can be easily

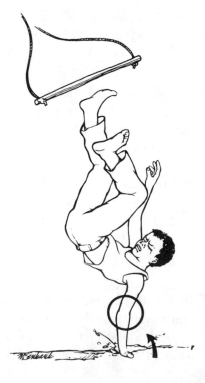

Figure 8.7 *Mechanism of elbow injuries.* (Reproduced by permission from Wilkins KE. Fractures and dislocations of the elbow region. In: Rockwood CA, Wilkins KE, King RE, eds. Fractures in children, 3rd ed. Philadelphia: JB Lippincott, 1991:694.)

missed. Radiographically, fracture lines may be difficult to detect, and a posterior fat pad sign may be the only evidence of fracture. Comparison views of the uninjured elbow may be necessary to differentiate between fracture lines and physeal growth plates. Generally these fractures require referral to an experienced orthopedic surgeon.

Both the medial and lateral condyles and epicondyles of the distal humerus are susceptible to fracture. The radiographic evaluation of these fractures can also be difficult owing to the variable presence of emerging ossification centers. Careful evaluation and occasionally an arthrogram can indicate whether surgical treatment is needed.

Fractures of radial head or proximal radial growth plate can be difficult to diagnose. The child usually comes to medical attention after a fall on an outstretched arm. There is mild swelling of the elbow and tenderness directly over the radial head. Pronation and supination of the forearm will also be painful. Radiographically, a posterior fat pad sign may be the only indication of an injury to the proximal radius.

Traumatic Dislocation of the Elbow

As children enter their second decade, the incidence of soft tissue injuries to the elbow increases. The most dramatic of these is the elbow dislocation. The mechanism usually involves a fall onto a hyperextended and abducted arm resulting in a dislocation of the radius and ulna in a posterior and lateral direction. Consequently, the medial collateral ligament is disrupted either as a ligament rupture or as an avulsion fracture of the medial epicondyle. The biceps, brachialis, and triceps insertions are usually intact. Gentle closed reduction is almost always successful. A relatively short period of immobilization of the elbow at 90° of flexion is the recommended treatment. Recurrent dislocation of the elbow is extremely rare.

Acute Injuries of the Adult Elbow

Anterior Capsular Sprains

In the adult athlete, soft tissue injuries around the elbow are more common than osseous injuries. The humerus, radius, and ulna serve as long lever arms for the elbow and consequently subject the elbow to large rotational forces. Hyperextension of the elbow from either a direct blow to the forearm or a fall onto an outstretched hand can cause a sprain of the anterior capsule. This seemingly minor injury may cause significant anterior elbow pain. As a result, the patient will tend to hold the elbow in a flexed position to relieve the stress on the anterior capsule. Unfortunately, this can lead to fibrosis of the capsule in a flexed position and loss of full elbow extension. Therefore, soon after the injury, range-of-motion exercises should be instituted to maintain full elbow extension. Nonsteroidal anti-inflammatory medications are helpful for decreasing the inflammation during the acute phase of the injury. If early return to activity is required, extension stop braces or taping can help prevent reinjury of the anterior capsule.

Traumatic Dislocation of the Elbow

In the adult, dislocation of the elbow is usually due to a hyperextension force. The tip of the olecranon is forced into the olecranon fossa on the posterior aspect of the humerus. This levers the coronoid process of the ulna beneath the trochlea of distal humerus, allowing the elbow to dislocate in a posterior direction. The articulation of the proximal radius and ulna usually remains intact (Fig. 8.8). Therefore

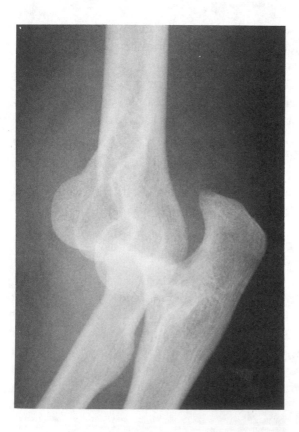

Figure 8.8 Radiograph of a traumatic elbow dislocation.

the radial head is also levered beneath the distal humerus and dislocates in a posterior direction. Thus in an elbow dislocation, both the ulnohumeral and radiocapitellar joints are disrupted. In addition to the capsular injury, the medial collateral ligament is almost always disrupted.

Intravenous sedation or sometimes general anesthesia is required to perform a gentle closed reduction of the elbow because the biceps, brachialis, and triceps muscles contract in response to the elbow dislocation. Although many techniques have been described, all generally apply distal traction to the forearm, pulling the coronoid process distal and anterior to the trochlea of the humerus, allowing for a gentle reduction. Again, the force of the biceps and brachialis anterior to the elbow and the force of the triceps posterior to the elbow provide stability to the reduced elbow.

If no associated injuries have occurred, early motion of the elbow is begun after the acute phase of the injury subsides. This is essential because scarring of the elbow capsule may lead to permanent loss of flexion and extension.

Medial Collateral Ligament Injuries

The medial collateral ligament can also be injured acutely in throwing sports. The elbow is subjected to large valgus forces during throwing. The athlete will complain of sudden onset of pain and often report feeling a "pop" on the medial aspect of the elbow during a delivery. The most common type of injury is an avulsion of the ligament from the medial epicondyle. This is followed in frequency by an avulsion from the ulnar insertion and then by a midsubstance rupture of the ligament. The type of injury can often be detected by palpation for the site of maximum tenderness. As the medial collateral ligament is the primary stabilizer of the elbow against valgus rotation, surgical repair of the acute injury is usually indicated in a throwing athlete.

Tendon Avulsions

A rupture of the distal biceps tendon is not an uncommon injury, although occurrence of this injury has never been reported in a female patient. The typical patient is an active male, 40 to 50 years of age. In 80% of the cases, the rupture occurs in the dominant extremity. The mechanism of injury is usually an eccentric action. That is, the biceps tendon is contracting vigorously while the muscle is being elongated by an extension force greater than the flexion or supination force generated by the muscle. On examination, there is a palpable defect

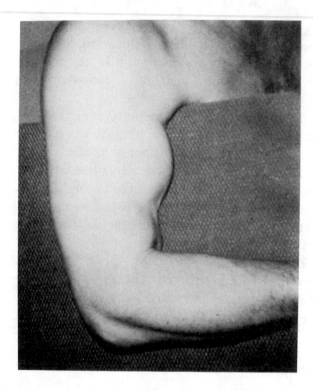

Figure 8.9 *Avulsion of the distal biceps tendon.* (Reproduced with permission from Coonrad RW. Tendonopathies at the elbow. In: Tullos HS, ed. Instructional Course Lectures 40. Park Ridge, IL: American Academy of Orthopaedic Surgeons, 1991:25–32.)

and ecchymosis in the cubital fossa. Upon activation of the biceps, there is a noticeable defect and bulge of the biceps muscle belly (Fig. 8.9). Treatment options are surgical and nonsurgical although most authors recommend surgical treatment. If treated nonoperatively, the biceps tendon will develop scar tissue to the deeper brachialis muscle. Loss of flexion strength will be minimal. However, the loss of supination strength will be significant. In an athlete or manual laborer, loss of supination strength is unacceptable and surgical treatment is indicated. The return of strength is much greater if the biceps tendon is repaired acutely. Even though retraction of the biceps muscle and tendon is present at late diagnosis, it is still possible to perform an anatomic repair, even 2 to 5 years after the injury.

Olecranon Bursitis

Acute olecranon bursitis causes a relatively painless superficial swelling of the posterior aspect of the elbow. It usually follows direct blunt trauma to the posterior elbow. If the bursitis is not infectious in nature, it can be treated with rest, protection, and anti-inflammatory medication. Aspiration of the bursa carries the risk of introducing infection or creating a fistula. If the bursa becomes chronically inflamed, surgical excision of the entire bursa is indicated.

Chronic Injuries of the Elbow

Repetitive stress on the elbow and its surrounding structures is extremely common in throwing athletes as well as in those involved in racquet sports. Chronic injuries of both elbow and shoulder are frequently seen as a result. This section will discuss the most common chronic elbow injuries in both children and adults.

Chronic Injuries of the Pediatric Elbow

Valgus Stress Syndromes

Elbow pain is a common complaint of adolescents participating in throwing sports, most notably baseball. Pain on the medial side of the elbow around the medial epicondyle is often referred to as "Little League elbow." This is a stress injury to the structures of the medial elbow secondary to tensile forces generated during the throwing motion (Fig. 8.10). Pain can be localized to the common flexor pronator muscle origin or the growth center of the medial epicondyle. Occasionally, radiographs will demonstrate fragmentation or widening of the medial epicondyle. Rest and a gradual return to activity are usually successful. If symptoms persist and activity is continued, an avulsion of the medial epicondyle may occur. If the fragment is markedly displaced or elbow instability is demonstrated, surgical treatment may be required.

Osteochondral Injuries

Lateral elbow pain is another common complaint of throwing athletes and gymnasts. During the acceleration phase of throwing, significant valgus forces are generated at the elbow. Consequently, the radiocapitellar joint is subjected to compressive forces while the medial side undergoes tensile forces. In gymnastics, landing on the hands with the arms fully extended also creates large compressive and valgus forces across the elbow (Fig. 8.11). These repeated compressive forces on the capitellum are believed to lead to avascular necrosis and, occasionally, osteochondral fractures of the capitellum.

Avascular necrosis, also referred to as osteochondritis dissecans, of the capitellum is a temporary loss of blood supply to the bone just

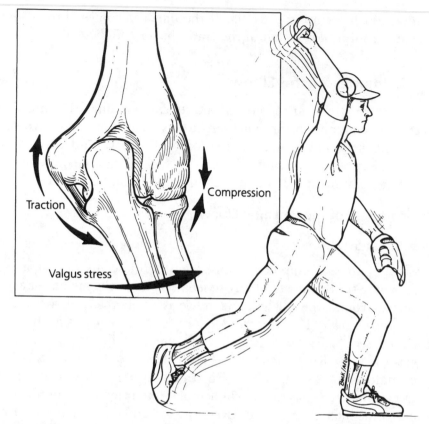

Figure 8.10 *Stresses generated around the elbow during throwing.*

beneath the articular cartilage. As this area of bone is revascularized and replaced with new immature bone, it is in a weakened state. As a result, it is at risk of microfractures and fragmentation when subjected to compressive forces. Therefore these patients complain of pain with activity, mild to moderate elbow swelling, and a loss of the last 10° to 20° of elbow extension. If no evidence of loose bodies in the elbow exists, restriction of activities will lead to a resolution of symptoms and a gradual return to activity. However, a history of a locked elbow or intermittent locking or sharp pain suggests the presence of a loose osteochondral fragment in the elbow joint. This requires arthroscopic surgical removal. Drilling of the base of the defect of the capitellum may be beneficial.

Chronic Injuries of the Adult Elbow

In the skeletally mature athlete, overuse injuries are common. The overuse syndromes present as joint problems, musculotendinous injuries, nerve entrapment, or a combination of any of these.

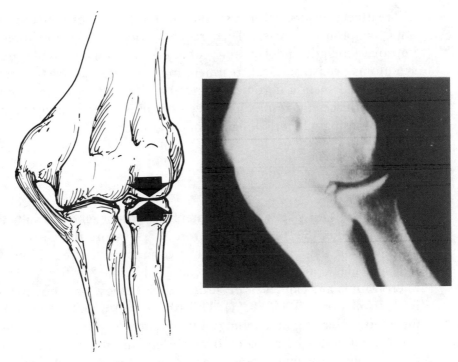

Figure 8.11 *Chronic valgus stresses leading to loose body formation.* (Reproduced by permission from Anderson TE. Anatomy and physical examination of the elbow. In: Nicholas YA, Harshmann EB, eds. The upper extremity in sports medicine. St. Louis: Mosby Year Book, 1990:329.)

Medial Collateral Ligament Injuries

Chronic injuries to the elbow are secondary to repetitive microtrauma to the articular cartilage, subchondral bone, joint capsule, and ligaments. Because most sports activities create a valgus force about the elbow, the medial-side injuries are due to tensile forces. The medial collateral ligament is the structure most commonly involved. Repetitive tensile loading of the ligament leads to microtears and eventual laxity. As a result, the athlete usually complains of pain along the medial elbow that is worse during the activity. On examination, tenderness is localized over the medial collateral ligament, distal to the medial epicondyle. Pain will be elicitied when valgus stress is applied to the elbow held in 20° to 30° of flexion. When compared with the other side, it may be possible to detect the increased laxity, and this can also be apparent on stress radiographs. Routine radiographs may demonstrate calcification within the medial collateral ligament or spur formation at the ulnar insertion of the medial collateral ligament.

Treatment begins with rest and anti-inflammatory medications until symptoms decrease. Then rehabilitation can be instituted to improve strength and flexibility of the supporting musculature. If symptoms persist, surgical treatment may be required. As the medial collateral ligament is chronically attenuated, direct repair may not be possible. Successful results have been obtained with ligament reconstruction using palmaris longus tendon grafts.

Osteochondral Injuries

During most sports activities, the lateral side of the elbow is subjected to compression due to the valgus forces. Therefore the capsule and ligaments on the lateral side are not commonly injured. However, the articular cartilage and subchondral bone suffer repetitive microtrauma and can result in chronic lateral elbow pain due to loose body formation (see Fig. 8.11). The athlete will usually complain of intermittent locking or catching of the involved elbow. On examination, crepitus can be palpated over the lateral elbow joint. Routine radiographs occasionally reveal the loose bodies, but an arthrogram obtained by computed tomography (CT) may be required to confirm their presence. Once detected, arthroscopic surgical removal of loose bodies is required. Postoperatively, attention is turned to regaining the range of motion and strength of the supporting musculature.

In addition to the valgus force generated during sports activities, the elbow is commonly driven into extension. This results in a forceful impact of the olecranon tip into the olecranon fossa on the posterior aspect of the distal humerus. This may lead to osteophyte formation on the tip of the olecranon or the walls of the olecranon fossa and subsequent painful block to full extension. On examination, there will be a firm mechanical block to full extension. In some cases the osteophytes may fracture and form loose bodies in the posterior aspect of the elbow. Again, radiographs or CT arthrography will confirm the presence of osteophytes and loose bodies.

Initial treatment is rest and anti-inflammatory medication as long as loose bodies are not creating mechanical symptoms. As pain subsides, treatment concentrates on regaining range of motion. If symptoms persist, arthroscopic surgical removal of osteophytes and loose bodies is indicated. Afterward, it is important to maintain the range of motion obtained by surgical debridement of the elbow.

Musculotendinous Injuries

Musculotendinous injuries are the most common elbow injuries in adult athletes. Lateral epicondylitis is an overuse injury of the common extensor muscles originating on the lateral epicondyle of the humerus (Fig. 8.12). This muscle group is susceptible to overuse injuries, especially in racquet sports, thus the term "tennis elbow." Surgical explorations have demonstrated that the extensor carpi radialis brevis tendon is the most commonly involved. In addition, electromyographic analysis of the forearm musculature during tennis ground strokes has shown the extensor carpi radialis brevis muscle to have the greatest activity. Primarily, the common extensor muscles act to stabilize the wrist during most athletic activities.

Lateral epicondylitis occurs equally in men and women and is most common during the fourth and fifth decades. Seventy-five percent of patients experience symptoms in the dominant arm. The patient complains of pain on the lateral side of the elbow that increases during sports activities. In addition, activities such as lifting or grasping for objects can elicit lateral elbow pain. On physical examination, tenderness is localized to the distal aspect of the lateral epicondyle.

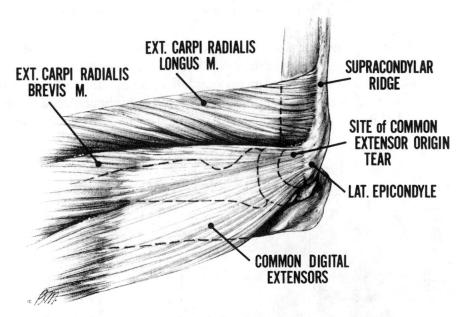

Figure 8.12 *Musculotendinous units involved in lateral epicondylitis.* (Reproduced by permission from Froimson AI. Tenosynovitis and tennis elbow. In: Green DP, ed. Operative hand surgery, 3rd ed. New York: Churchill Livingstone, 1993:2001.)

Resisted wrist extension is often painful. Passive volar flexion of the wrist can cause pain near the lateral epicondyle, especially when the wrist is pronated and the elbow is extended. Radiographs of the elbow are usually normal; however, calcification within the soft tissues around the lateral epicondyle may be detected in up to 25% of patients.

Ninety percent of patients with lateral epicondylitis recover with nonsurgical treatment. In the early stages, rest and anti-inflammatory medication may entirely relieve symptoms. With increasing duration of symptoms, other modalities may be required to obtain relief. Especially for those involved in racquet sports, equipment changes may be helpful. A change in racquet handle size or weight may prove beneficial. The use of a counterforce brace (Fig. 8.13), also referred to as a tennis elbow strap, may allow the athlete to participate in activities with minimal symptoms. The circumferential band is placed around the proximal forearm and secured tightly enought to apply pressure over the proximal common extensor musculotendinous junction. Conceptually, this distal pressure relieves some of the tensile stresses at the common extensor muscle origin at the lateral epicondyle. In conjunction, a rehabilitation program of stretching and strengthening will often lead to a resolution of symptoms.

For patients with recalcitrant cases, injections of corticosteroids may be necessary to relieve pain. The injections are often successful if followed by a rehabilitation program of strengthening and stretching. However, steroid injections carry the risk of subcutaneous atrophy and skin changes, and repeated injections will lead to a significant

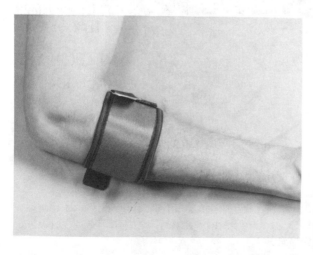

Figure 8.13 *Counterforce brace applied to the proximal forearm for treatment of lateral epicondylitis.*

weakening of the tendon. Therefore no more than three injections are recommended.

Finally, if the forms of treatment described above prove unsuccessful, surgical treatment is indicated. Surgical techniques range from debridement of the extensor carpi radialis brevis tendon to complete release of the common extensor origin. Again, therapy to improve flexibility and strength is important for a successful result.

Inflammation of the common flexor pronator origin, or medial epicondylitis, can be a source of medial elbow pain. The pronator teres and flexor carpi radialis are the most commonly involved tendons in this process. This syndrome is most common in activities that create valgus stress in the elbow and involve repetitive wrist flexion such as pitching, tennis, and swimming, although it is often referred to as "golfer's elbow." Medial epicondylitis is reportedly 7 to 20 times less common than lateral epicondylitis. Medial epicondylitis is equally prevalent among men and women and is most common in the fourth and fifth decades of life. Surgical treatment is rarely necessary as treatment with rest, stretching, and strengthening is often successful. The counterforce brace is helpful in some cases but is not as reliable as in cases of lateral epicondylitis. Corticosteroid injections may be beneficial in troublesome cases. If symptoms persist despite rest and rehabilitation, other sources of the pain should be sought. Incompetency of the medial collateral ligament or entrapment of the ulnar nerve may be the cause of pain in recalcitrant cases.

Tendinitis of the triceps tendon posteriorly or the biceps and brachialis tendon anteriorly is not seen as often as medial and lateral epicondylitis. However, the treatment protocols are similar, and rest, anti-inflammatory medication, and rehabilitation usually lead to resolution of the symptoms.

Nerve Entrapment Syndromes

Nerve entrapment syndromes around the elbow are antoher source of pain in the athlete with repetitive demands on the upper extremity. The ulnar nerve may become chronically inflamed in its course posterior to the medial epicondyle and around the posterior aspect of the elbow joint (Fig. 8.14). This is especially true in activities that involve repetitive elbow flexion or direct trauma to the posterior elbow. In the early stages the athlete will complain of a vague pain in the posterior medial elbow. Tinel's sign will be positive over the course of the ulnar nerve, especially where it is subcutaneous. The pain may radiate into

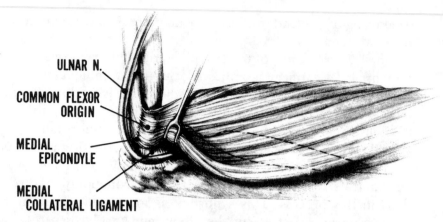

ULNAR N.

COMMON FLEXOR
ORIGIN

MEDIAL
EPICONDYLE

MEDIAL
COLLATERAL LIGAMENT

Figure 8.14 *Relation of the ulnar nerve to the muscles and ligament of the medial elbow.* (Reproduced by permission from Froimson AI. Tenosynovitis and tennis elbow. In: Green DP, ed. Operative hand surgery, 3rd ed. New York: Churchill Livingstone, 1993:2002.)

the forearm and the fourth and fifth fingers. The athlete may report subluxation of the ulnar nerve from the groove during activites that involve elbow flexion, and this is detectable on physical examination. Awakening at night with paresthesias into the hand is not uncommon. In later stages, sensory changes in the fourth and fifth fingers may become apparent. Motor weakness can be detected as atrophy of the hypothenar eminence of the hand or intrinsic muscle atrophy in the hand. Electrodiagnostic studies such as electromyography (EMG) or nerve conduction studies can be helpful in confirming the diagnosis.

In the early stages, rest and anti-inflammatory medication are beneficial. If nighttime awakening is a problem, splinting of the elbow or placing a pad in the antecubital fossa will prevent elbow hyperflexion during sleep and, therefore, relieve the stress on the ulnar nerve. If symptoms persist or sensory or motor deficits become apparent, surgical treatment is indicated. Rarely a case is successfully treated by only a release of the fascia overlying the ulnar nerve. Anterior transposition of the ulnar nerve, in which the nerve is taken out of its groove and permanently placed anterior to the elbow joint, is the usual surgical procedure.

Radial nerve entrapment can be the source of lateral elbow pain. This is especially true in suspected cases of lateral epicondylitis that do not respond to treatment. Although referred to as radial nerve entrapment, the pathology is usually at the level where the radial nerve has bifurcated into the posterior interosseous nerve and the radial sensory nerve. Unfortunately, diagnosis of radial nerve entrapment is difficult to confirm. Entrapment may result in pain in the region of the common extensor muscles that is exacerbated in activities that involve forced wrist extension. In other cases, pain may not be a predominant symptom, but weakness will be quite apparent. The athlete will display weakness of the extensors of the wrist, fingers, and thumb. Electrodiagnostic studies often do not provide evidence of nerve entrapment. Therefore pain relief by injections of lidocaine into the area of the posterior interosseous nerve may be required to confirm the diagnosis.

Rest, anti-inflammatory medication, and rehabilitation are usually successful in resolving the symptoms. In protracted cases, surgical exploration and release of the radial tunnel may be required to alleviate the nerve entrapment.

Rehabilitation

In general, rehabilitation of the injured elbow involves treatment of an acute injury or an acute exacerbation of a chronic injury. The goals are to maintain or improve range of motion, to recover or improve muscular strength, and to return to the preinjury activity level. This section will discuss the general approach to elbow rehabilitation. Further information can be found in Chapter 5.

Acute Injuries

Acute injuries usually come to medical attention during the inflammatory phase of recovery. Rest, ice, compression, and elevation constitute the standard treatment protocol during this phase. Cryotherapy delays but does not eliminate inflammation and, owing to vasoconstriction, prevents the extension of hematoma. In addition, the application relieves pain by slowing nerve impulses and decreasing muscle spasm. The most efficient way to apply cold therapy is with ice packs, ice massage, or ice baths. Nonsteroidal anti-inflammatory medications will also help decrease the cell-mediated response to the acute injury. By decreasing the inflammatory response, pain and swelling are diminished, allowing for earlier rehabilitation.

Following the short inflammatory phase, the body begins to repair injured tissue. During this reparative phase physical therapy and rehabilitation are begun. Foremost is maintaining range of motion. The elbow, especially in the adult, has a propensity to develop contractures even after minor injuries. Therefore, as soon as symptoms permit, therapy should concentrate on regaining full extension and flexion. Although the extremes of motion are not necessary for activities of daily living, a lack of full extension may render an athlete unable to perform at preinjury levels. Active motion and passive stretching in flexion, extension, pronation, and supination will help prevent posttraumatic joint contractures. However, overaggressive stretching is not recommended in the early phases because of the risk of bone formation within the muscle, this is called *myositis ossificans*. This can lead to marked stiffness. At the same time, muscle strengthening should be instituted. Because the medial flexor pronator group and the lateral extensor group serve as stabilizers of the elbow, regaining strength is an important component of full recovery. Once nearly full range of motion is painless and muscle strength exceeds 90% of normal, it is safe for the athlete to return to active participation. A gradual return will allow for muscle retraining and help prevent reinjury of the elbow.

Both cold and heat are fundamental modalities used to treat injuries. The benefits of cryotherapy have been discussed above and these extend into the reparative phase of the injury. Heat relieves pain by diminishing nerve impulses, improves blood supply by vasodilatation, and increases enzymatic and metabolic rates. In addition, heat increases collagen extensibility and decreases muscle tone and spasm.

Ultrasound therapy has the ability to quickly raise the temperature of deeper tissues. This high-frequency vibrational energy also produces mechanical effects such as increased cell permeability, improved diffusion of ions, and diminished scar formation. The technique of phonophoresis uses this improved diffusion to deliver medications such as salicylates and corticosteroids to the deeper muscles.

Several other local modalities exist for treatment of soft tissue injuries. Transcutaneous electrical nerve stimulation (TENS), electrogalvanic stimulation, and continuous passive motion are only a few of the widely used techniques. Although reports of excellent treatment results with these modalities exist, there is little scientific evidence to support their use.

Chronic Injuries

In the acute presentation of a chronic injury, the early treatment is the same as for an acute injury. Once the acute phase has passed, attention must be turned to prevention of recurrent injuries. Many chronic injuries are due to lack of flexibility, muscle weakness, poor mechanics, or a combination of these. In addition, training schedules and equipment selection should be evaluated.

Flexibility of the entire upper extremity is important for normal elbow function. Limited range of motion of the shoulder necessitates compensation at the elbow to achieve desired hand positions. Therefore active motion and passive stretching should include the shoulder girdle, shoulder, elbow, wrist, and hand.

Muscle strengthening should concentrate on improving endurance as well as strength. Most overuse injuries of the elbow involve some component of muscular fatigue. Isometric and low-weight, high-repetition exercises for all directions of elbow motion are the initial phase of muscle rehabilitation. As with flexibility, the shoulder, wrist, and hand strength and endurance must also be improved because deficits will have an effect on the elbow. As strength and endurance increase, high-intensity and eccentric exercises may be added to the treatment protocol. Training aids such as elastic bands, pulleys, dumbbells, and computerized feedback systems are commonly used in rehabilitation protocols. Supervision to ensure proper technique and progress will avoid the unnecessary setbacks of reinjury.

The final component of a successful recovery is improved mechanics during the desired activity. Minor changes in mechanics, such as a change in pitching motion, arm position during vaulting, or forearm position during ground strokes, can significantly alter the stresses placed on the elbow. Coaches and trainers are often instrumental in detecting the subtle alterations in performance mechanics and helping the athlete to correct them.

With improved flexibility, strength, and mechanics, the athlete should gradually return to full activity. Once back, it is important to maintain these three components to prevent the nuisance of reinjury.

Differential Diagnosis of Elbow Pain

Acute Pain

- ✗ Dislocation
- ✗ Fracture
- ✗ Sprain (medial collateral ligament complex)
- ✗ Biceps tendon rupture
- ✗ Anterior capsular sprain

Chronic Pain

Medial Elbow Pain

- ✘ Medial epicondylitis ("golfer's elbow")
- ✘ Medial valgus overload (medial collateral ligament)
- ✘ Ulnar nerve entrapment

Lateral Elbow Pain

- ✘ Lateral epicondylitis ("tennis elbow")
- ✘ Radial nerve entrapment
- ✘ Osteochondral injury (radiocapitellar joint)

Suggested Readings

Andrews JR, Craven WM. Lesions of the posterior compartment of the elbow. Clin Sports Med 1991;10(3):637–652.

Coonrad RW. Tendonopathies at the elbow. Instr Course Lect 1991;40:17–24.

Curl WW. Office treatment of elbow injuries in the athlete. Instr Course Lect 1994;43:55–61.

Glousman RE. Ulnar nerve problems in the athlete's elbow. Clin Sports Med 1990;9(2):365–377.

Hoppenfeld S. Physical examination of the spine and extremities. Norwalk, CT: Appleton-Century-Crofts, 1976:35–57.

Hotchkiss RN. Common disorders of the elbow in athletes and musicians. Hand Clin 1990;6(3):507–515.

Jobe FW, Ciccotti MG. Lateral and medial epicondylitis of the elbow. J Am Acad Orthop Surg 1994;2(1):1–8.

Jobe FW, Kvitne RS. Elbow instability in the athlete. Instr Course Lect 1991;40:17–24.

Morrey BF. The elbow. Philadephia: WB Saunders, 1985.

Nicholas JA, Hershman EB. The upper extremity in sports medicine. St. Louis: CV Mosby, 1990:273–362.

CHAPTER **9**

Hand and Wrist Injuries

Lisa R. Reznick

In general, hand and wrist injuries comprise approximately 25% of all athletic injuries. The risk of injuries depends on the type of sport, with those who play sports requiring physical contact or direct ball-handling being the most vulnerable. However, athletes may also incur some of the same injuries by a fall onto an outstretched hand.

In contact sports such as football and hockey, players are exposed to a multitude of acute hand and wrist injuries. For example, ligament ruptures, joint dislocations, tendon avulsions, and fractures are commonly associated with these sports. Volleyball, basketball, and baseball players may sustain similar injuries secondary to direct contact with the ball, lunging for the ball, or sliding into base. In other sports such as gymnastics, however, athletes are more susceptible to chronic injuries secondary to the repetitive motions required to perform their routines. Repetitive motion is also common in baseball, golf, tennis, and other racquet sports, with potential development of problems such as tendinitis and carpal tunnel syndrome secondary to the cumulative effects of the repetitive stress.

Because of the prevalence of hand and wrist injuries, those who initially evaluate the injured athletes, such as coaches, trainers, and physicians, must be able to differentiate those injuries that are easily treated from those that require referral to a specialist. Improperly treated or misdiagnosed injuries can result in loss of function, deformity, degenerative arthritis, and possible permanent disability.

The purpose of this chapter is not only to discuss common athletic hand and wrist injuries but also to assist in their diagnosis, treatment, and referral. For a better understanding of these injuries and their subsequent treatment, a brief overview of the hand and wrist anatomy will be covered. The remainder of the chapter will discuss various athletic hand and wrist injuries ranging from acute to chronic disorders.

Anatomy

The anatomy of both the wrist and the hand is intricate and complex. It is beyond the scope of this chapter to cover every detail of the anatomy. The discussion will focus on the joint, ligament, and tendon anatomy.

Ligament and Joint Anatomy

The wrist joint is formed by the radius, ulna, and carpus (Fig. 9.1). Rotation of the forearm occurs primarily in the radioulnar compartment of the wrist joint, whereas flexion and extension of the wrist occurs in the radiocarpal compartment. The carpus consists of eight carpal bones (see Fig. 9.1) that are tightly connected together with

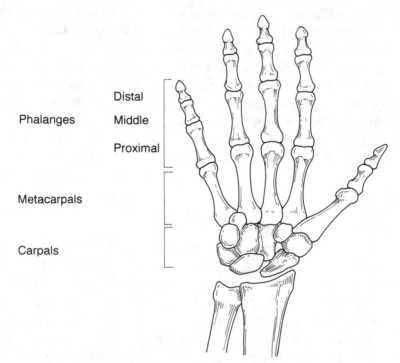

Figure 9.1 *Bones of the hand and wrist.*

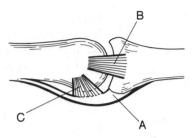

Figure 9.2 *Interphalangeal joint anatomy with volar plate (A), collateral ligament (B), and accessory collateral ligament (C).*

intercarpal ligaments. Only very limited motion is possible between carpal bones. The carpals form joints with the metacarpals, which are therefore called carpometacarpal joints. Distally, the carpals form metacarpophalangeal joints with the proximal phalanx. Except for the thumb, which has two, each finger has three phalanges, and therefore each has a proximal interphalangeal (PIP) and distal interphalangeal (DIP) joint. Both metacarpophalangeal and interphalangeal joints allow only flexion and extension and are guided by medial or radial and lateral or ulnar collateral ligaments. On the volar or palm side of the DIP and PIP joints, a cartilaginous shelf called the volar plate inserts onto the base of the most distal phalanx (Fig. 9.2). This volar plate adds significant stability to the joint and serves as an attachment point for the collateral ligament complex (see sections below on joint and ligament injuries).

Extensor Tendons

A review of the anatomy of the extensor and flexor tendons will assist the examiner in evaluating the injured athlete's hand. The function of the hand and fingers relies on the intricate balance of these tendons.

The extensor tendons of the wrist, thumb, and fingers are located in separate compartments at the level of the wrist (Fig. 9.3). The thumb extensor tendons include the abductor pollicis longus and extensor pollicis brevis. The radial and ulnar wrist extensors, the main finger extensors (extensor digitorum communis), and accessory index and little finger extensor tendons make up the remaining tendons.

The main finger extensors proceed distally across the dorsum of the hand en route to their respective fingers. Just proximal to this level, transverse tendinous bands (juncturae tendinae) interconnect the extensor tendons of the long, ring, and little fingers. Through this interconnection, these bands can allow complete extension of the long, ring, or little finger despite a complete laceration of one of the main extensor tendons proximally. Therefore careful examination of

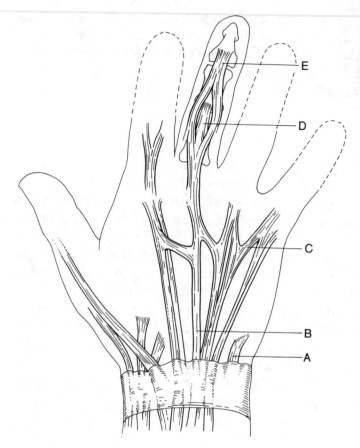

Figure 9.3 *Extensor tendon anatomy of hand and wrist with wrist extensors (A), finger extensors (B), junctura (C), central slip (D), and terminal slip (E).*

each individual digit is necessary to avoid false-negative findings of this type.

Over the distal half of the proximal phalanx, the extensor tendon divides into three slips, including the central slip flanked by the two lateral slips of the terminal extensor tendon. After merging with the medial bands of the interosseous tendons, the central tendon inserts onto the dorsal base of the middle phalanx. The central tendon functions to extend the proximal interphalangeal joint. If the central tendon is compromised, extension of the PIP joint will be affected.

The terminal extensor tendon is formed over the middle phalanx where the lateral bands of the extensor tendon unite with the corresponding lateral divisions of the interosseous tendons. Therefore disruption of the terminal extensor tendon results in the inability to extend the DIP joint.

Flexor Tendons

For each digit, there are two separate tendons that act to bend the finger, the flexor digitorum superficialis (FDS) and the flexor digitorum profundus (FDP). The thumb's anatomy is different and relies on the flexor pollicis longus and flexor pollicis brevis for bending.

In the forearm, the independent FDS tendons are superficial to the conjoined FDP tendons. At the level of the wrist, the flexor tendons of the fingers and the flexor pollicis longus tendon of the thumb travel through the carpal tunnel with the median nerve.

Traversing the palm, the flexor tendons to each corresponding finger maintain the relation of the FDS superficial to the FDP tendon. Both tendons then become contained within a tight tunnel, extending from about the level of the metacarpophalangeal joint to the midportion of the middle phalanx.

Over the proximal phalanx, the relation of the FDS and FDP tendons changes (Fig. 9.4). The FDS tendon splits into two slips, allowing the FDP tendon to pass through the FDS tendon and become more superficial. The slips of the FDS tendon then insert into the midportion of the middle phalanx and function to flex the PIP joint. The FDP tendon continues its course to insert into the base of the distal phalanx. The FDP is a strong flexor tendon that primarily functions to flex the DIP joint but also contributes to flexion of the PIP joint. Therefore, with a laceration of only the FDS tendon, the patient will still be able to weakly flex the PIP joint.

For the thumb, the flexor pollicis brevis originates in the palm and inserts onto the base of the proximal phalanx to flex the metacarpophalangeal joint. As described above, the flexor pollicis longus travels through the carpal tunnel and inserts onto the base of the thumb's distal phalanx. Similar to the FDP tendon of the fingers, the flexor pollicis longus primarily bends the distal thumb joint but also contributes to bending the metacarpophalangeal joint.

Tendon Injuries

Sports participation exposes athletes to the risk of sustaining certain soft tissue injuries of the hand and wrist. Among these disorders, tendon injuries are possible and sustained secondarily to direct contact with the game ball or other players. Both flexor and extensor

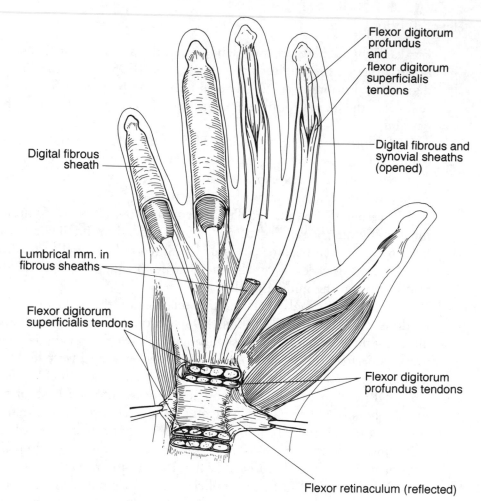

Flexor digitorum
profundus
and
flexor digitorum
superficialis
tendons

Digital fibrous and
synovial sheaths
(opened)

Digital fibrous
sheath

Lumbrical mm. in
fibrous sheaths

Flexor digitorum
superficialis tendons

Flexor digitorum
profundus tendons

Flexor retinaculum (reflected)

Figure 9.4 *Flexor tendon anatomy of the hand and wrist.*

tendons are equally at risk. The most common injuries include jersey
finger, mallet finger, and boutonniere deformity. These injuries require a thorough physical examination for prompt diagnosis and
proper treatment.

General Evaluation

Open and closed injuries are evaluated similarly. However, if the
injury is associated with an open wound, the initial step is thorough
irrigation of the site with normal saline or other sterile solution.
In general, lacerations or wounds should alert the examiner to
the possibility of an associated tendon laceration, fracture, or joint
dislocation.

Tendon injuries are difficult to evaluate and frequently can be misdiagnosed. Therefore a careful, thorough examination of the hand is essential to diagnose these injuries. In addition, each finger must be examined individually.

The finding most indicative of a tendon injury is an alteration in the natural attitude or posture of the hand. Normally, the posture of the hand is formed by a cascade of flexed fingers, gradually increasing from the index to small finger (Fig. 9.5). However, with a flexor tendon injury, the normal cascase is disrupted and the involved digit is held in more extension. In the case of an extensor tendon rupture or laceration, the unsupported finger flexes more than in the usual cascade because of the unopposed actions of the FDS and FDP tendons.

Physical examination involves manually testing the function of all tendons to each finger. In general, with a complete tendon laceration or rupture, total function will be lost. However, if the tendon is partially lacerated, the athlete may still be able to maintain motion but will experience pain and weakness when tested against resistance.

The extensors of the fingers and thumb are examined by placing the patient's hand on a flat surface and having the patient independently lift each digit off of the table. In addition, the continuity of these tendons can be demonstrated through the tenodesis effect. If the tendons are intact, passive wrist extension will flex the fingers, whereas passive wrist flexion will extend the fingers. Therefore, if an

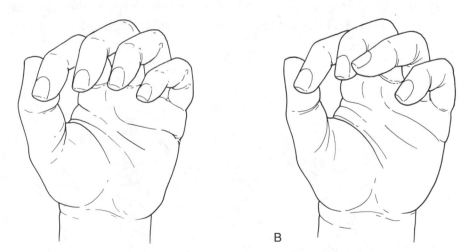

A   B

Figure 9.5 *Normal finger cascade (A) and abnormal cascade owing to flexor tendon rupture (B).*

extensor tendon is disrupted, the finger will not extend with passive wrist flexion.

Examination of the flexor tendons requires isolating the function of the FDS and FDP. FDP function can be demonstrated by stabilizing the PIP joint in extension while the patient actively bends the tip of the finger (Fig. 9.6). FDS function is isolated by stabilizing the other fingers in extension and having the patient actively bend the unblocked finger (Fig. 9.7). By keeping the other fingers extended, the contribution of the FDP tendon to PIP joint flexion is prevented.

Jersey Finger

Avulsion of the FDP tendon from its insertion is a relatively common injury in athletes. This injury is referred to as jersey finger, because it typically occurs when a player tries to impede or tackle an opponent by grabbing the person's jersey. During this type of maneuver, the player's actively flexed finger becomes forcibly extended as the opponent attempts to escape. The ring finger is most frequently affected.

Unfortunately, this injury is often misdiagnosed as a "jammed finger" and, consequently, improperly treated. Accurate diagnosis is based on the mechanism of injury and a detailed examination. Initially, a delay in diagnosis may occur because the athlete can still flex the finger's PIP joint through an intact FDS tendon. Therefore, to an inexperienced eye, the inability to flex the DIP joint may go undetected. As previously described in this chapter, the function of the FDS and FDP tendons should be tested independently to avoid this error.

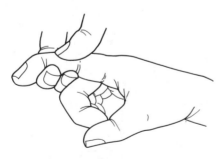

Figure 9.6 *Testing flexor digitorum profundus tendon function.*

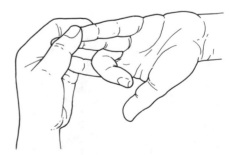

Figure 9.7 *Testing flexor digitorum superficialis tendon function.*

Other than the loss of active DIP joint flexion, clinical findings may include a tender mass in the palm as well as swelling and ecchymosis of the finger. The mass is the retracted FDP tendon and is usually located at the level of the distal palmar crease. Thorough evaluation includes radiographs of the injured finger. These x-rays may assist in the diagnosis. Occasionally, a bony fragment from the distal phalanx may be avulsed with the tendon. When not associated with an avulsion fracture, the ruptured tendon can retract freely through its sheath and into the palm. By retraction into the palm, the tendon's complex blood supply becomes completely disrupted. In this case, the tendon must be surgically repaired within 7 to 10 days of onset to avoid tendon necrosis and contracture. Therefore prompt referral of these injuries to a specialist is strongly recommended.

Following surgery and sufficient tendon healing, the patient will require extensive hand therapy to regain motion and strength before returning to play.

Mallet Finger

Mallet or "baseball" finger is a common tendon injury among athletes. Athletes participating in ball-handling sports such as baseball, basketball, and football are particularly at risk. The most frequent mechanism of injury entails forced flexion of the DIP joint of an actively extended finger. This longitudinal force disrupts the terminal extensor tendon from its insertion onto the distal phalanx. This mechanism occurs most commonly when a player's fingertip is forced into flexion by direct contact with the ball. Similar to FDP tendon ruptures, these injuries can be associated with a bony avulsion from the dorsal base of the distal phalanx. Lacerations over the dorsum of the DIP joint also can disrupt the extensor mechanism and lead to a mallet digit.

These injuries, like FDP tendon ruptures, are frequently misdiagnosed as a "jammed finger." Mallet finger refers to the clinical posture of the digit resulting from disruption of the terminal extensor tendon. The tip of the finger droops into flexion, and the patient is unable to actively extend the DIP joint (Fig. 9.8). Furthermore, tenderness, swelling, and ecchymosis of the DIP joint may be present. Radiographs of the finger should be obtained to diagnose an associated avulsion fracture of the distal phalanx.

Unlike FDP tendon ruptures, the majority of mallet fingers can be treated nonoperatively. Early management is necessary to preserve function and prevent deformity. Treatment requires continuous dorsal splinting of the DIP joint in full extension for 6 to 8 weeks. The splint should not include the PIP joint, which is allowed to move freely. The splint can be fashioned from alumiform, orthoplast, or moleskin-covered metal.

Application of the splint demands a strategic technique of taping. The initial piece of tape is placed longitudinally on the volar aspect of the finger and pulled over the tip of the finger and top of the splint. The second and third pieces are placed perpendicular to the first and circumferentially around the middle of the distal and middle phalanges, respectively (Fig. 9.9). With the splint in place, many athletes can continue to participate in practice and sports as tolerated.

Following the primary treatment period, the finger should be splinted intermittently for another 6 to 8 weeks. The splint should be worn during sports participation and at night. When the splint is not being worn, gentle active range-of-motion exercise of the DIP joint is encouraged.

Certain circumstances mandate referral to a specialist for surgical treatment. The situations include tendon avulsions associated with fractures involving more than 50% of the articular surface of the distal phalanx or subluxation of the DIP joint. In these cases, open reduction with internal fixation of the avulsed fragment is strongly recommended. Formal hand therapy is prescribed following adequate tendon healing.

Boutonniere Deformity

Boutonniere deformity is a postural deformity of the finger resulting from an imbalance of forces between the flexor and extensor mechanisms. There are usually three component to a boutonniere deformity: PIP joint flexion, DIP joint hyperextension, and occasional metacarpophalangeal joint hyperextension (Fig. 9.10).

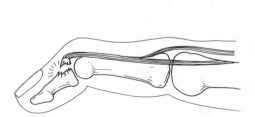

Figure 9.8 *Typical appearance of a mallet finger.*

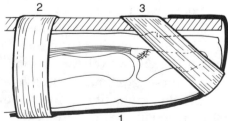

Figure 9.9 *Splinting technique for a mallet finger by placing tape in position 1 first, followed by 2 and 3.*

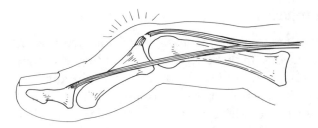

Figure 9.10 *Boutonniere deformity of the finger.*

In general, the common etiology of boutonniere deformity is damage to the central extensor tendon. In acute closed injuries, the characteristic boutonniere deformity may not be present initially and usually develops over a period of 10 to 21 days following injury. For this reason, early diagnosis and treatment of these injuries are important. Physical findings may include a painful, swollen, and tender PIP joint. There is either loss of active extension or weakened PIP joint extension against resistance. The flexion deformity of the PIP joint is secondary to the loss of the central slip function and the unopposed force of the FDS. Disruption of the central slip allows the lateral bands to migrate volar to the axis of the PIP joint, causing further flexion of the PIP joint and extension of the DIP joint.

Prompt treatment of these injuries is required to prevent permanent PIP and DIP joint contractures and scarring. Early treatment focuses on continuous immobilization of the PIP joint in full extension, excluding the DIP joint, for 6 to 8 weeks. Several three-point-type devices are available for treatment. These splints immobilize the PIP by a three-point configuration and allow the DIP joint to actively flex and extend (Fig. 9.11).

Following the initial treatment period, the player should wear the splint intermittently for another 6 to 8 weeks. The splint should be worn during practice and play.

If the boutonniere deformity is chronic, initial treatment remains similar to that for the acute injury. However, failure of the deformity to improve may necessitate surgical treatment.

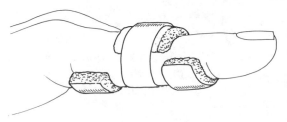

Figure 9.11 *Three-point splint for a boutonniere deformity.*

Fingertip and Nailbed Injuries

Injuries to the fingertip are one of the most common acute hand problems. Various structures may be involved including the skin, subcutaneous tissue, bone, nail, and nailbed. The cause in approximately 25% of cases is compression between two objects.

To recognize the severity of these injuries and understand their treatment, one must be familiar with the anatomy of the fingertip and nailbed. The nailbed, comprising the germinal and sterile matrixes, is the soft tissue located beneath the nail and is responsible for nail production and growth (Fig. 9.12). The germinal matrix produces 90% of the nail, and the sterile matrix, which adheres to the underlying periosteum of the distal phalanx, contributes 10%. The base of the nail fits into the nail fold, which is a recess with a floor of germinal matrix and a roof covered by the nail wall. As a thin extension of the nail wall, the eponychium attaches to the base of the nail while the paronychium is the soft tissue extending along the lateral borders of the nail. Just beyond the eponychium, the lunula or white arc of the nail marks the junction of the germinal and sterile matrixes. The lunula serves as a helpful landmark in clinically assessing the involvement and severity of injury to the germinal and sterile matrixes.

Trauma to a fingertip can cause an array of injuries ranging from a simple subungual hematoma to a complex laceration or tip amputation. A careful physical examination will allow one to determine the severity of the injury and the involved structures.

Subungual Hematoma

Trauma to a nailbed can cause the germinal or sterile matrix to bleed. Bleeding from a nailbed laceration can dissect between the nail and

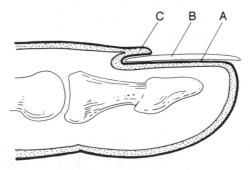

Figure 9.12 *Anatomy of the nailbed with nailbed (A), nail (B), and eponychium (C).*

the nailbed and produce a subungual hematoma. Clinically, the hematoma can appear as a dark red to black discoloration underneath the nail. Because this blood is under pressure, the patient experiences throbbing pain. If the hematoma involves less than 25% of the visible nail surface, then the laceration is probably small. In this case, the subungual hematoma can be decompressed using a large sterile needle or heated paper clip to penetrate the nail and allow the blood to drain. However, if more than 25% of the nail is involved, then a more extensive laceration is probably present and it should be evaluated for a possible surgical repair. If left untreated, the nailbed laceration can result in permanent deformity of the nail. When treating these injuries, refrain from removing the nail, because this can further damage the germinal and sterile matrixes if performed improperly.

Nailbed Lacerations

Nailbed lacerations should be suspected in patients who sustain significant trauma to the fingertip or nail. If there is a bleeding laceration involving the nail or a large subungual hematoma, then there is evidence of involvement of the underlying nailbed. Careful inspection of the nailbed is important. In addition, a significant nailbed injury may be indicative of an associated distal phalanx or tuft fracture. Therefore radiographs of the involved finger should be obtained to exclude a fracture. If a fracture is present, then proper splinting and occasionally percutaneous pinning may be required to stabilize the fracture and aid in soft tissue healing.

A lacerated nail matrix should be treated after careful removal of the nail and under controlled, sterile conditions using a finger tourniquet. Therefore, when a severe nailbed laceration is suspected, prompt referral is recommended. However, the initial evaluator should perform preliminary irrigation and placement of a clean, moist dressing.

Crush, Avulsion, and Fingertip Amputations

These injuries are complex and require careful examination followed by irrigation and debridement of the wound. If the wound is contaminated, then antibiotics and tetanus prophylaxis are also recommended. Bleeding can be controlled with elevation of the extremity above heart level, application of a pressure dressing, and direct pressure over the wound. If a portion of soft tissue was avulsed from the fingertip, the piece should be rinsed off thoroughly, wrapped in a moistened towel, and placed in a plastic bag. This avulsed tissue may be able to serve as a skin graft in repairing the soft tissue.

The vast majority of open fingertip injuries can be treated with closure of lacerations and dressing changes to areas with lost skin. Very acceptable results are obtained by allowing new skin to grow in from the edges of the uncovered areas. This new skin, however, will remain sensitive for a long time. Occasionally, the area without skin is large or deep enough to require some type of skin graft. The decision regarding treatment should be made by a physician with experience in treating these injuries.

Joint and Ligament Injuries

Because the wrist and hand conmprise 22 bones and numerous joints, the ligaments of the hand and wrist play a crucial riole in maintaining stability during the use of the hand. Ligament injuries therefore result in immediate disability and require meticulous evaluation and treatment. This section will discuss the most common ligament injuries in the hand and wrist.

Proximal Interphalangeal Joint Dislocations

Among the sports-related hand injuries, PIP joint dislocations are common. Specifically, dorsal dislocations of the PIP joint are the most common dislocation of the hand. These injuries occur primarily in ball-handling and contact sports. Dependent on the mechanism of injury, the PIP joint can also be dislocated laterally or volarly. Radiographs of the injured digit are critical for diagnosis, detection of associated fractures, and assistance with treatment (Fig. 9.13).

Dorsal dislocations occur secondary to an axial load that hyperextends the PIP joint, rupturing the insertion of the volar plate. This volar plate rupture may be associated with an avulsion fracture from the base of the middle phalanx. Following volar plate rupture, the middle phalanx displaces dorsally or posterior to the proximal phalanx.

Clinically, the player presents a diffusely swollen, tender, ecchymotic, and deformed finger. If the radiographs indicate either a pure dislocation or only a small avulsion fracture, then closed reduction can be attempted. The reduction manuever requires slight accentuation of the hyperextension deformity and application of gentle longitudinal traction. If a large or comminuted fracture exists, then

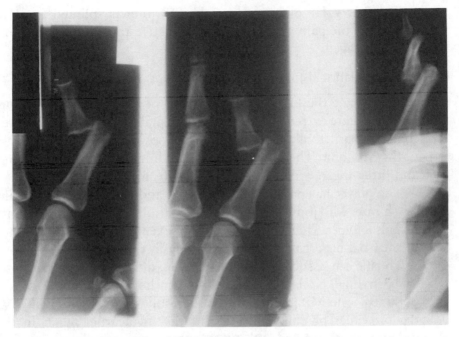

Figure 9.13 *X-rays of proximal interphalangeal and distal interphalangeal joint dislocations.*

referral to a specialist for treatment of this complex injury is encouraged.

Following reduction, joint stability should be documented by both active and passive range of motion. In addition, postreduction radiographs should confirm joint congruency and exclude other fractures. Postreduction immobilization involves splinting the PIP joint in 20° to 30° of flexion for 1 to 3 weeks. Buddy-taping to the adjoining digit is then implemented until the athlete achieves full, pain-free range of motion.

Volar Plate Injuries

Rather than frank dislocation, hyperextension of the PIP joint may cause damage to only the volar plate. The volar plate usually ruptures from its distal attachment and may be associated with a small avulsion fracture from the base of the middle phalanx.

The player frequently has a painful, swollen digit with tenderness and ecchymosis primarily located on the volar aspect of the PIP joint. Radiographs of the digit may appear normal or show a small chip fracture volar to the PIP joint.

To treat volar plate injuries, the PIP joint is splinted for 1 to 2 weeks. As the pain gradually resolves, active range of motion should be encouraged.

Metacarpophalangeal Joint Dislocations

In contrast to the PIP joint, dislocations of the metacarpophalangeal (MP) joint are extremely rare. Athletes usually sustain these injuries in football, basketball, baseball, or soccer secondary to hyperextension of the MP joint. The border digits, including the thumb, index finger, and little finger, are most commonly affected.

The player has pain, diffuse swelling, and ecchymosis of the finger or thumb MP joint. In dorsal dislocations, physical examination reveals a hyperextended MP joint and flexed PIP joint. The prominent metacarpal head can be palpated easily in the palm.

To rule out associated fractures of the metacarpal head or base of the proximal phalanx, radiographs of the injured finger must be obtained. The MP joint is most commonly dislocated dorsally, with the proximal phalanx posterior to the metacarpal head. In those dislocations associated with a large intra-articular fracture, referral to a specialist is recommended.

For dislocations not associated with a fracture or associated with only a small avulsion fragment, closed reduction can be attempted. However, closed reduction becomes increasingly difficult with each subsequent attempt. Therefore the first reduction maneuver must be performed properly. With the wrist in flexion, the maneuver initially entails accentuation of the deformity by hyperextending the proximal phalanx. Next, the examiner administers gentle, longitudinal traction on the digit while simultaneously manipulating the proximal phalanx over the metacarpal head.

Following reduction, joint congruency is confirmed and other fractures are excluded radiographically. The majority of these joints are stable and can be treated with buddy-taping until full, pain-free range of motion is attained. Occasionally MP dislocations are complex and irreducible by closed means. If initial adequate attempts at closed reduction are not successful, a complex dislocation should be suspected. These cases should be referred to a hand specialist.

Gamekeeper's Thumb

Gamekeeper's or skier's thumb refers to a common ligamentous injury of the thumb's metacarpophalangeal joint. Although it is associated with skiing, all athletes are susceptible to this injury. The common mechanism is radial deviation or an abduction force to the extended MP joint of the thumb, causing a partial or complete rupture of the ulnar collateral ligament.

Because of the precarious nature of this injury, early diagnosis and treatment is necessary. Improper treatment can cause untoward results such as chronic instability and arthritis. Therefore distinguishing between partial and complete ruptures of the ulnar collateral ligament is crucial. For example, sprains or incomplete ruptures can be treated with cast immobilization. However, complete ruptures require referral to an orthopedist and subsequent surgical intervention. Thorough knowledge of the anatomy of the thumb MP joint will assist in evaluation and proper management of these injuries.

The collateral ligaments are composed of two components, the proper and accessory ligaments, which originate from the thumb metacarpal head and insert into the ulnar base of the proximal phalanx and the volar plate, respectively (see Fig. 9.2). These components provide lateral support and prevent volar subluxation of the joint. In flexion, the accessory ligament relaxes while the proper ligament tightens to stabilize the joint. In contrast, the accessory ligament becomes taut in extension and provides the majority of joint stability. Therefore both components of the collateral ligament must be competent to support the MP joint throughout the entire range of motion. The abduction stress test, a diagnostic maneuver discussed below, is designed to evaluate the integrity of each of these components.

These injuries occur secondary to a sudden, forced radial deviation of the thumb MP joint due to a fall onto an outstretched hand or during contact with the ball or another player. Physical examination reveals diffuse ecchymosis and swelling of the thumb with more discrete tenderness of the MP joint ulnarly.

Definitive diagnosis of a complete tear is based on evaluation of MP joint stability. The abduction stress test, performed with radial deviation of the thumb MP joint in full extension and in slight flexion, assesses the integrity of the accessory and proper ligaments, respectively. In comparison to the opposite thumb, a complete tear exists if the injured MP joint deviates ulnarly more than 30° with this maneuver (Fig. 9.14).

Before stress examination, however, radiographs of the thumb MP joint must be obtained to rule out fractures. If fractures are present, stress examination of the MP joint may displace these fractures and create further instability. Undisplaced fractures can be treated with a

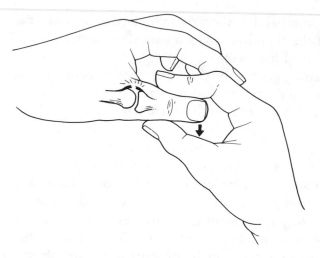

Figure 9.14 *Testing for a tear of the ulnar collateral ligament of the thumb metacarpophalangeal joint.*

short arm thumb spica cast for 4 to 6 weeks; however, displaced fractures may have to be treated operatively to prevent chronic instability of the MP joint.

For clinically stable joints without deviation on provocative testing, treatment entails protective thumb spica splinting or casting until resolution of pain. In casting these injuries, position the thumb in adduction to prevent further stress to the ulnar collateral ligament. Partial ruptures with mild instability are treated with 4 to 6 weeks of thumb spica immobilization, followed by active flexion and extension exercises.

Conversely, complete ruptures must be recognized acutely and may have to be surgically repaired by a specialist. With complete ruptures, the adductor pollicis aponeurosis may become interposed between the torn ligament and its insertion site, creating a Stener lesion. In this situation, anatomic healing of the ulnar collateral ligament is impossible without operative intervention. To avoid the surgical complexity and inferior results associated with chronic ruptures, prompt recognition and expedient referral of ulnar collateral ligament injuries is essential.

Radial Collateral Ligament Injuries

This injury is analogous to gamekeeper's thumb, but is 10 times less common and involves the radial collateral ligament of the thumb MP joint. The ligament is injured by a sudden ulnarly deviated or adduction force to the thumb MP joint.

Physical evaluation of the player's thumb will reveal swelling, ecchymosis, and radial tenderness of the MP joint. The guidelines for diagnosis and treatment of partial and complete ruptures of the radial collateral ligament are similar to those previously described for injuries to the ulnar collateral ligament.

Scapholunate Dissociation

Wrist injuries are common in sports. Usually, these injuries occur secondary to a single traumatic episode such as a fall onto an out-stretched upper extremity.

Unfortunately, serious ligamentous injuries of the wrist are frequently misdiagnosed as simple "sprains." In general, evaluation of wrist injuries should carry a high index of suspicion for ligamentous ruptures and subsequent instability.

Specifically, in scapholunate dissociation, the ligament between the scaphoid and lunate bones is partially or completely disrupted. This disruption impairs the functional stability between the scaphoid and lunate bones and alters wrist kinematics.

Diagnosis of this injury can be challenging. Physical examination may reveal point tenderness of the scapholunate joint, located just distal to Lister's tubercle. In addition, anteroposterior and lateral radiographs of the wrist may demonstrate an abnormal alignment between the scaphoid and lunate bones.

Because of the complexity of this injury, prompt referral to a specialist for definitive diagnosis and treatment is highly recommended. Failure of early identification and treatment of scapholunate dissociations can result in progressive degenerative arthritis and significant, permanent disability.

Fractures

Although this chapter is primarily dedicated to soft tissue injuries of the hand, fractures of the phalanges and metacarpals are not uncommon in sports. Despite their prevalence, these fractures are frequently misdiagnosed, resulting in permanent deformity and functional impairment. Prompt recognition and proper treatment of these injuries is paramount to ensure motion and prevent deformity.

In general, intra-articular fractures require anatomic reduction of the articular surface to prevent loss of motion and arthritis. Fractures that result in malrotation or malalignment of the digit require manipulation and stabilization, with possible internal fixation and immobilization. In particular, spiral and oblique fractures of the metacarpals and phalanges must be critically evaluated for rotational deformity. Displaced and unstable fractures are treated

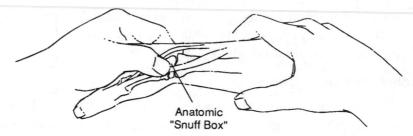

Anatomic
"Snuff Box"

Figure 9.15 *The anatomic snuff box.* (Reproduced by permission from Richmond J, Shahady E. Sports medicine for primary care. Cambridge, MA: Blackwell Science, 1995.)

with reduction, possible internal fixation for stabilization, and immobilization.

Carpal fractures can occur in contact as well as noncontact sports. Frequently misdiagnosed as "wrist sprains," these injuries require a thorough examination and a high index of suspicion for early recognition and proper treatment. Early treatment is essential, especially in the case of scaphoid fractures, which are notorious for problematic healing. If treated improperly, carpal fractures can result in such complications as delayed union or nonunion, malunion, pain, stiffness, deformity, and degenerative arthritis. The three most common carpal fractures associated with sports are of the scaphoid, hamate, and trapezium bones.

The scaphoid is the most commonly fractured carpal bone. The injury usually involves a fall onto an outstretched hand. The player usually complains of radial-sided wrist pain that is exacerbated with wrist extension or gripping motions. Examination may reveal swelling over the dorsoradial aspect of the wrist. Classically, these fractures are diagnosed by point tenderness dorsally, deep within the anatomic snuff box located between the first and third extensor compartments. This area can be palpated just distal to the radial styloid (Fig. 9.15). Further workup of these fractures involves a complete set of radiographs including a scaphoid series.

Chronic Overuse Injuries

Repetitive motions in sports subject athletes to overuse injuries or tendinitis. Tendinitis refers to an inflammatory process of the tendon sheaths. Although any flexor or extensor tendon may be involved, certain wrist tendons are anatomically more prone to tendinitis than others.

Clinically, the athlete complains of pain either after or during activity. With palpation, the localized area is usually warm, swollen, tender, and possibly crepitant. Upon physical examination of the affected tendons, pain is exacerbated with resisted motion and passive stretch.

In general, the initial treatment of tendinitis includes conservative measures such as rest, immobilization, and nonsteroidal anti-inflammatory drugs (NSAIDs). The majority of these cases can be successfully managed by nonoperative means.

De Quervain's Tenosynovitis

Stenosing tenosynovitis is commonly localized to the region of the radial styloid. In this area, the tendons of the abductor pollicis longus and extensor pollicis brevis traverse the styloid en route to their insertions into the thumb. Symptoms of de Quervain's disease primarily include pain and swelling. This pain may be localized or radiate proximally into the forearm or distally into the thumb. These symptoms are exacerbated with activities requiring thumb adduction and flexion and wrist ulnar deviation.

Clinically, athletes can present with prominence of the soft tissue overlying the radial styloid. Crepitance of the tendons may be palpated in this region. On physical examination, resisted thumb abduction and extension may aggravate the patient's discomfort. Finkelstein's test, performed with thumb adduction and ulnar deviation of the wrist, typically reproduces the symptoms (Fig. 9.16). However, because Finkelstein's test is nonspecific, the diagnosis of de Quervain's disease should not be based solely on this finding.

Treatment consists of limiting activities by immobilization in a splint for 3 to 6 weeks and administration of NSAIDs. When these measures fail, injection of corticosteroid into the first dorsal compartment is often attempted. In recalcitrant cases, surgical release of the first dorsal compartment is required.

Wrist Flexor and Extensor Tendinitis

The wrist has a pair of wrist extensor tendons and flexor tendons. Wrist flexion is accomplished through a radial and ulnar flexor tendon (flexor carpi radialis and ulnaris). Wrist extension is similarly powered by a radial and ulnar extensor (extensor carpi radialis longus and extensor carpi ulnaris). The radial wrist extension has another extensor, the extensor carpi radialis brevis. Virtually all of the tendons can be affected by excessive repetitive motion and develop a

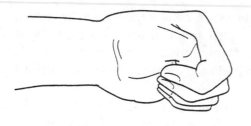

Figure 9.16 *Finkelstein's test.* (Reproduced by permission from Gross J, Fetto J, Rosen E. Musculoskeletal examination. Cambridge, MA: Blackwell Science, 1995.)

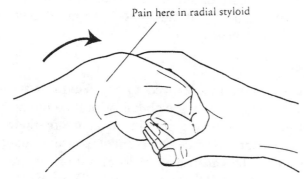

Pain here in radial styloid

tendinitis-like picture. This results in local pain and tenderness directly over the affected tendon. The athletes complain of pain during and after use of the hand and wrist. Occasionally, swelling due to inflammation of the tendon can be seen. In severe cases some crepitus can be felt with use of the affected tendon.

The treatment approach is similar to that for all cases of overuse tendinitis. Relative rest with avoidance of the offending motion is usually obtained by a temporary wrist splint. Icing and NSAIDs are used to decrease the pain and swelling. Once the intial pain and swelling have subsided, stretching exercises are started. If symptoms allow, this is progressed to strengthening exercises of the involved muscle-tendon units. Return to activites must be gradual to avoid flare-ups. In resistant cases a local corticosteroid injection around the tendon can be attempted. Surgery is rarely needed.

Entrapment Neuropathies

The median, radial, and ulnar nerves are the three main peripheral nerves that provide the sensation and motor nerves to the hand and wrist. In the forearm and wrist these nerves follow a complex course around muscles, tendons, and bony structures. Along this course they are susceptible to entrapments by the surrounding structures. Pressure on a peripheral nerve can cause chronic pain in the distribution of that nerve. If the entrapment is severe or prolonged, actual numbness and muscle weakness can develop. Two of the most common entrapment neuropathies will be discussed in this section.

Carpal Tunnel Syndrome

Sports requiring repetitive, forceful gripping such as golf, racquetball, and tennis subject participants to the development of carpal tunnel syndrome. Sustained wrist positions of extreme extension and flexion also can result in compression of the median nerve at the wrist.

The carpal tunnel is a confined space at the level of the wrist, containing nine flexor tendons and the median nerve. If this canal's volume is compromised by either tendon or synovial inflammation, anomalous lumbrical muscles, or a space-occupying lesion, the median nerve will become compressed.

Players primarily complain of numbness and tingling in the radial three and a half digits, corresponding to the sensory distribution of the median nerve. In addition, these symptoms may be exacerbated at night, awakening the player from sleep.

Findings on clinical examination include a positive Phalen's test and Tinel's sign and altered sensation in the median nerve distribution. Phalen's test is performed by having the player extend the elbows and maximally flex the wrists. This manuever compresses the median nerve by increasing the intracompartmental pressure of the carpal tunnel. This test is positive if tingling develops in the median nerve distribution within 1 minute of wrist flexion. Tinel's sign is positive if tapping volarly over the carpal tunnel reproduces the tingling.

A thorough sensory evaluation includes light touch, pin prick, and two-point discrimination. Of these three tests, two-point discrimination is the most sensitive. The ability to detect two points of a paper clip or caliper to within 5 mm on the pads of the median innervated digits constitutes a normal study. Clinical comparison with the opposite hand is essential.

Chronic compression can affect the motor function of the median nerve. Late clinical findings may reveal weakness and atrophy of the thenar musculature. The player may demonstrate decreased grip strength or relay a history of dropping objects.

The clinical diagnosis can be verified by electrophysiologic tests. These studies also can identify other areas of compression as well as involvement of other nerves.

Initial treatment of carpal tunnel syndrome entails conservative measures including neutral wrist splints, rest, and NSAIDs. In addition, corticosteroid injections into the carpal tunnel can decrease inflammation and, in turn, relieve compression of the median nerve. For players with persistent symptoms despite conservative therapy, referral to a specialist for surgical decompression of the carpal tunnel is recommended.

Ulnar Tunnel Syndrome

Although less common than carpal tunnel syndrome, ulnar tunnel syndrome refers to compression of the ulnar nerve within Guyon's canal at the wrist. Bordered by the hamate and pisiform bones, Guyon's canal is a confined space containing the ulnar nerve and artery. Ulnar nerve entrapment can result from blunt trauma to the hypothenar eminence, pisotriquetral arthritis, or fractures of the hamate or pisiform bones. In cyclists, ulnar nerve or "handlebar" palsy can occur from leaning with this area on the handlebars.

Clinically, athletes can have signs and symptoms related to ulnar sensory and motor functions. Players commonly experience paresthesias in the ulnar sensory distribution to the pads of the ulnar one and a half digits. Sensory function can be assessed by two-point discrimination. In addition, ulnar motor function may be impaired, resulting in weakness of pinch and grip. The ulnar nerve innervates the interossei, hypothenar, and adductor pollicis muscles. Interossei function can be tested by either resisted spreading of the patient's fingers or the ability to move the extended long finger independently from side to side. Again, clinical diagnosis can be confirmed by electrophysiologic studies.

Treatment depends on the etiology of the patient's ulnar tunnel syndrome. Conservative treatment is similar to the protocol described above for carpal tunnel syndrome. Usually, "handlebar" palsy can be resolved with rest, adjustment of seat and handlebar height, and use of cushioned handlebars and padded gloves.

Differential Diagnosis of Hand or Wrist Pain

Acute Finger or Thumb Pain

✗ Dislocation of metacarpophalangeal, proximal interphalangeal, or distal interphalangeal joint

✗ Gamekeeper's thumb or mallet finger
✗ Jersey finger
✗ Boutonniere injury
✗ Fracture

Wrist Pain

Acute Pain

✗ Gamekeeper's thumb
✗ Dislocation
✗ Scapholunate dissociation
✗ Carpal fracture (scaphoid)
✗ Radius fracture

Chronic Pain

✗ Wrist flexor-extensor tendinitis
✗ De Quervain's disease
✗ Carpal tunnel syndrome
✗ Ulnar tunnel syndrome
✗ Unrecognized scaphoid fracture
✗ Unrecognized ligament injury (gamekeeper's thumb, schapolunate dissociation)
✗ Arthritis

Suggested Readings

Burton RI, Eaton RG. Common hand injuries in the athlete. Orthop Clin North Am 1973;4:809–838.

Green DP. Operative hand surgery. 3rd ed. New York: Churchill Livingstone, 1993.

Isani A. Prevention and treatment of ligamentous sports injuries to the hand. Sports Med 1990;9(1):48–61.

Kahler DM, McCue FC. Metacarpophalangeal and proximal interphalangeal joint injuries of the hand including the thumb. Clin Sports Med 1992;11(1):57–76.

McCue FC, Meister K. Common sports hand injuries. Sports Med 1993;15(4):281–289.

Newland CC. Gamekeeper's thumb. Orthop Clin North Am 1992;23(1):41–48.

Pitner MA. Pathophysiology of overuse injuries in the hand and wrist. Hand Clin 1990;6(3):355–364.

Rettig AC. Hand injuries in football players (soft tissue trauma). Phys Sportsmed 1991;19(12):97–107.

Rettig AC. Closed tendon injuries of the hand and wrist in the athlete. Clin Sports Med 1992;11(1):77–99.

Strickland J, Rettig AC. Hand injuries in athletes. Philadelphia: WB Saunders, 1994.

CHAPTER **10**

Injuries of the Thoracic and Lumbar Spine

William L. Craig III and Timothy N. Taft

The prevalence of soft tissue injuries of the thoracic and lumbar spine suffered during athletic participation is difficult to determine. Most injuries occur during practice or training, not during competition when health care providers are likely to be present. Furthermore, most athletes do not report minor injuries, which include a significant number of thoracolumbar spine injuries. Finally, most of these injuries are self-limiting and resolve without any formal treatment or without loss of time from practice or competition. It is estimated, however, that spine injuries account for some 10% to 15% of all sports-related injuries and are therefore not infrequently seen by coaches, trainers, and physicians. Proper diagnosis and treatment of these injuries is essential. Improper diagnosis and failure to recognize potentially serious injuries can lead to disastrous outcomes.

To safely and accurately diagnose and treat injuries to the thoracic and lumbar spine in athletes, it is necessary to (1) have a good general understanding of the normal anatomy of the thoracolumbar spine, (2) be able to perform a thorough and accurate examination of the thoracic and lumbar spine, recognizing potentially serious findings, (3) understand the pathophysiology of the more common injuries and how it relates to treatment, and (4) understand when the athlete is safe to return to practice or competition or when referral to a specialist is indicated. In this chapter, we will attempt to review the relevant anatomy and physical examination of the thoracic and lumbar spine, explain the pathophysiology of soft tissue injuries, review treatment modalities, and set guidelines for return to athletic participation or referral to a specialist.

Anatomy of the Thoracic and Lumbar Spine

The Vertebrae

The thoracic and lumbar spine consists of 12 thoracic and 5 lumbar vertebrae. They are named and numbered from proximal to distal T1 through T12 and L1 through L5. The vertebrae of the thoracolumbar spine have the same general shape and function (Fig. 10.1). However, there is some variation as one proceeds from the first thoracic to the fifth lumbar vertebra. Each vertebra can be divided into anterior and posterior elements. The anterior element of each vertebra is the vertebral body. The overall configuration of each body is that of a short cylinder. The thoracic vertebral bodies are heart-shaped and increase in size from T1 to T12 as they descend down the spine. In contrast, the lumbar vertebral bodies are larger and heavier than those of the thoracic spine and are wider in their transverse diameter than anteroposteriorly. The last three lumbar vertebral bodies are wedge-shaped, having a greater height anteriorly than posteriorly when viewed laterally.

Attached to the posterior aspect of the vertebral bodies are the posterior elements or the vertebral arch. The vertebral arch is composed of two pedicles and two laminae that unite to form a partial circle. The space within this circle constitutes, when numerous vertebrae are placed one on top of the other, the spinal or vertebral canal. The spinal canal contains the spinal cord and the exiting spinal nerves. Multiple projections that serve as attachments for muscles and

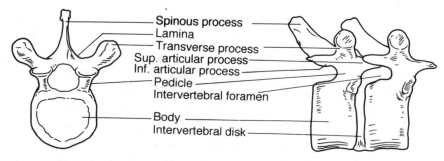

Spinous process
Lamina
Transverse process
Sup. articular process
Inf. articular process
Pedicle
Intervertebral foramen
Body
Intervertebral disk

Figure 10.1 *General anatomy of thoracic and lumbar vertebrae.* (Redrawn by permission from Hollinshead WH, Rosse C. Textbook of anatomy, 4th ed. Philadelphia: Harper & Row, 1985:287.)

ligaments as well as articulations extend from the posterior elements of the vertebral body. Two transverse processes project laterally from the junction of the lamina and the pedicles, and the spinous process projects posteriorly from the point at which the two laminae meet. As mentioned above, these serve primarily as attachments for ligaments and muscles. Because of the location of the pedicles on the vertebral bodies when they are stacked one on top of another, a notch remains between the inferior aspect of one pedicle and the superior aspect of the pedicle below. This opening is an intervertebral foramen that allows room for the spinal nerves to leave the spinal cord.

The vertebrae articulate through the intervertebral disks (discussed below) and the articular processes. Two superior articular processes project upward from the upper border of each lamina, and two inferior articular processes project downward from the lower border of each lamina. The superior articular processes of one vertebra articulate with the inferior articular processes of the vertebra immediately superior, forming a facet joint. The orientation of these facet joints allows for the range of motion in the thoracolumbar spine. In the thoracic spine these joints are positioned chiefly in the coronal plane. The articular surface of a superior articular process faces posteriorly, and the articular surface of the inferior process faces anteriorly. This position allows for side-to-side bending in the thoracic spine. However, the facet joints of the lumbar spine are oriented such that the superior articular process faces medially and the inferior articular process laterally, or in the sagittal plane. This orientation allows for flexion and extension in the lumbar spine.

Intervertebral Disks

The intervertebral disks serve as the main connection between the vertebral bodies. They provide a strong link between adjacent vertebrae while still allowing for movement. The disks may vary slightly in size and shape throughout the thoracolumbar spine; however, the organization of each disk is the same. Each disk is divided into two parts: a strong outer component, the annulus fibrosis, and an inner component, the nucleus pulposus (Fig. 10.2). The annulus fibrosis is made of fibrocartilage. Its fibers are organized in concentric rings with the fiber orientation of each ring rotated approximately 90°. Its main function is to withstand the stresses of the vertebral column and to contain the compressed nucleus pulposus. The nucleus pulposus consists of a mucoid viscoelastic material that acts as a shock absorber. This material is 70% to 90% water.

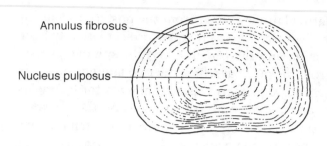

Annulus fibrosus

Nucleus pulposus

Figure 10.2 *Structure of an intervertebral disk.*

Muscles and Ligamentous Structures

Several muscular and ligamentous structures originate and attach to the thoracic and lumbar spine. They serve to stabilize the spine, as well as to allow for movement. The ligaments of the thoracolumbar spine can also be divided into anterior and posterior elements. There is one chief anterior ligamentous structure, the anterior longitudinal ligament (Fig. 10.3). This broad band of connective tissue located on the anterior and anterolateral surfaces of the vertebral bodies tends to limit spine extension.

There are several posterior spinal ligaments (see Fig. 10.3). The posterior longitudinal ligament runs on the posterior surface of the vertebral bodies within the spinal canal. The supraspinous ligament runs over the spinous processes for the entire length of the thoracolumbar spine. The interspinous ligaments connect the low border of one spinous process with the upper border of another spinous process, with its most superficial edge blending with the supraspinous ligament. The most important posterior ligamentous

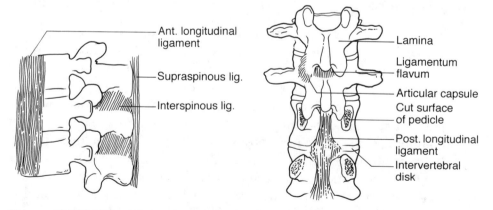

Ant. longitudinal ligament
Supraspinous lig.
Interspinous lig.
Lamina
Ligamentum flavum
Articular capsule
Cut surface of pedicle
Post. longitudinal ligament
Intervertebral disk

Figure 10.3 *Ligaments in and around the spine.* (Redrawn by permission from Hollinshead WH, Rosse C. Textbook of anatomy, 4th ed. Philadelphia: Harper & Row, 1985:295.)

structures are the ligamenta flava. They are paired ligaments located between adjacent lamina. These ligaments help to stabilize the spine in flexion. Finally, there are intertransverse ligaments that connect adjacent transverse processes.

The musculature of the back is arranged in multiple layers (Fig. 10.4). The true muscles of the back are covered by the muscles of the shoulders (trapezius, rhomboids, latissimus dorsi) and ribs (serratus posterior). The muscles of the thoracic and lumbar spine generally run in a longitudinal direction with multiple levels of origins and insertions. However, for the purpose of this chapter, it is not necessary to discuss each individual origin and insertion.

The superficial muscle layer is composed of the trapezius and the latissimus dorsi. The trapezius originates from the spinous processes

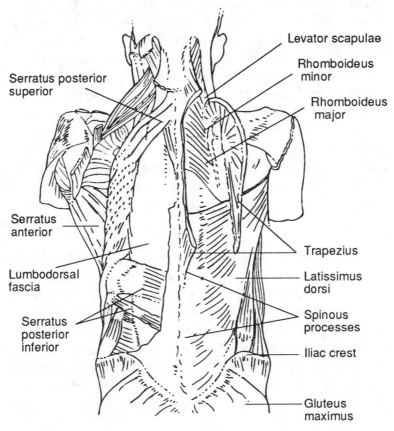

Figure 10.4 *Superficial muscles of the back and spine.* (Reproduced by permission from Richmond J, Shahady E. Sports medicine for primary care. Cambridge, MA: Blackwell Science, 1995.)

of the cervical and thoracic vertebrae, extends laterally, and inserts into the scapula. The latissimus dorsi originates from the spinous processes of the more inferior thoracic and the lumbar spine and extends superolaterally to insert on the scapula and humerus. Beneath the trapezius and latissimus dorsi, but superficial to the true musculature of the back, is the serratus posterior. The serratus posterior originates from the spinous processes and inserts onto ribs.

Beneath the serratus is the fascia that overlies the true muscles of the back. For the purpose of this discussion, we will divide the musculature of the back into the erector spinae and transversospinalis complex (Fig. 10.5). The erector spinae complex is the largest mass of muscle of the back and is composed of three separate muscles (iliocostalis, longissimus, and spinalis). It originates from the sacrum, iliac crest, and the spinous processes of the lumbar and the last two thoracic vertebrae. There are multiple areas of insertion on the ribs and on the transverse and spinous processes of the thoracic and lower cervical spine. The principal action of the erector spinae complex is to extend the spine as well as to provide support. The transversospinalis muscle complex, composed of the semispinalis, multifidi, and rotator muscles, lies deep to the erector spinae complex. These muscles generally originate from the transverse processes and insert onto the spinous processes. They usually span only one or a few vertebrae. The majority of the true muscles of the back are innervated by the dorsal rami of the spinal nerves, although some are innervated by the ventral rami.

Spinal Nerves

The spinal nerves or nerve roots leave the spinal cord in the spinal canal. Particularly in the lumbar spine, they travel for some distance in the spinal canal before they exit through the neural foramen. They are named and numbered relative to the vertebra under which they lie. Therefore there are 12 thoracic, 5 lumbar, and 5 sacral nerve roots. For example, the L5 root exits underneath the neural arch of the fifth lumbar vertebra. Once the roots have exited they become a complex plexus that eventually gives off the peripheral nerves such as the sciatic and femoral nerves.

History and Physical Examination

A thorough history and physical examination are essential when treating injuries of the thoracic and lumbar spine. More importantly,

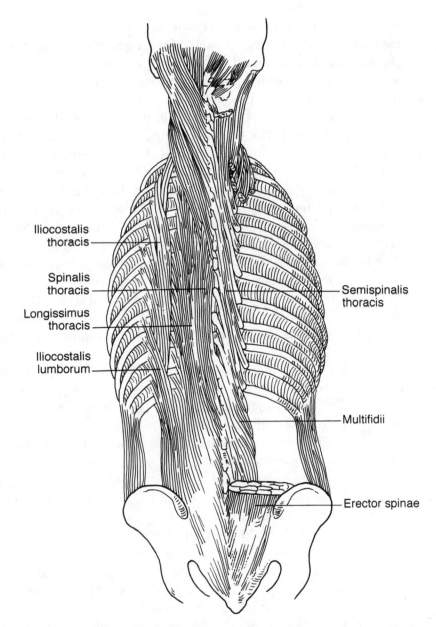

Figure 10.5 *Deep, true muscles of the spine.* (Redrawn by permission from Hollinshead WH, Rosse C. Textbook of anatomy, 4th ed. Philadelphia: Harper & Row, 1985:312.)

one should never be rushed or under any time constraints when examining an athlete with a back injury, especially an acute injury. If there is any concern that the injury is serious and may include neurologic damage, the athlete should be properly immobilized and examined immediately by a physician.

It is important to obtain an accurate and complete history of current illness with any back injury or pain. This information often leads directly to the correct diagnosis. In the majority of cases, the athlete's chief complaint is back pain, either acute or chronic. It is important to develop a thorough understanding of the pain. Where is it located? What is its character? What activities or movements exacerbate it? Also of importance in the history is the timing of events surrounding the onset of the pain. Even in chronic injuries the athlete tends to look for an acute event that was associated with the onset of the symptoms. However, the magnitude of the injury is often less than would be expected for the symptoms. One should determine if there was a direct blow associated with the onset of the pain. The presence or absence of neurologic symptoms should be documented.

After one has a good understanding of the history surrounding the injury, a thorough directed examination should be performed. The examination should include inspection, palpation, range-of-motion testing, and a neurologic assessment.

An initial inspection of the injured spine should be performed. One should view the patient from the back, as well as the side, to get an impression of the curvature of the spine. It is important to note any excessive lordosis or kyphosis of the spine, as well as side bending. It is also important to note the ease with which the patient ambulates and stands from a seated position. The athlete's ability to perform each movement can be helpful in determining the severity of the injury. After a complete inspection, one should palpate the entire thoracolumbar spine for areas of tenderness. From the history of present illness, one should have a general idea of the location of maximal tenderness. It is advisable to begin palpation away from the area of suspected injury and work toward it. The presence or absence of tenderness over the spinous processes should be documented. Any point tenderness should alert the examiner to the possibility of a fracture or bony contusion. In addition, tenderness or spasm of the paraspinal musculature should be noted. The sacroiliac joints, sciatic notches, and posterior thighs should also be palpated for tenderness.

After the anatomic location of maximal tenderness has been noted, the range of motion of the thoracolumbar spine should be tested. The normal range of motion of the thoracolumbar spine varies with individuals. In general, normal forward flexion, which occurs predominantly in the lumbar spine, is between 40° and 60° and extension is between 20° and 35°. Side bending, which occurs predominantly in the thoracic spine, is approximately 20° to the right and left. Rotation, which also occurs predominantly in the thoracic spine, is normally 90° in either direction. Documentation of the range of motion and any deviation from the normal range, asymmetry, or pain with movement should be noted. Pain with forward flexion is usually nonspecific; however, pain with extension can often be attributed to pathology of the facet joints or other posterior structures, such as pars interarticularis or the neural foramina. Also, pain with side bending or rotation may help to further delineate which muscle is injured or suspected of injury on the basis of history and palpation.

A thorough neurologic examination is necessary in evaluating thoracic and lumbar spine injuries when there is concern of spinal cord injury based either on the mechanism of injury or on the history. This should include a sensory examination of the thoracolumbar area and a sensory and motor examination of the lower extremities.

The neurologic examination of the thoracic spine is somewhat difficult. Sensation can best be tested using light touch over the thorax and abdomen (Fig. 10.6). Interpretation can often be difficult owing to the overlapping dermatomes in the area. Motor examination of the musculature can also be difficult. Paraspinal muscles are innervated by spinal nerves from several levels, and it is virtually impossible to determine the absence of one specific root. In addition, the motor examination is often limited because of the athlete's pain or muscle spasm.

An accurate neurologic examination of the lower extremities is essential in any athlete with a significant injury to the lumbar spine. Gross examination of the lower extremity muscle strength can be accomplished by asking the patient to perform a deep knee bend, toe walk, and heel walk. Any difficulty standing from the deep knee bend suggests quadriceps weakness. The inability to toe walk may represent gastrocnemius or soleus weakness, while difficulty in heel walking suggests weakness in ankle dorsiflexion. Following gross examination, specific muscle groups should be tested. This is best accomplished with the patient in the seated position with the legs hanging off the edge of the examination table. Specific muscle groups

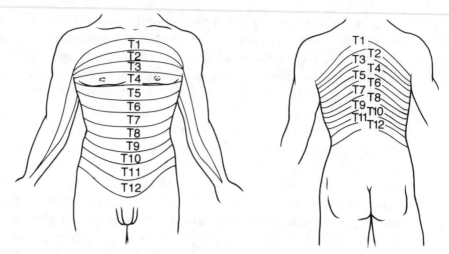

Figure 10.6 *Dermatomal distribution by spinal nerve of the chest and abdomen.* (Redrawn by permission from DeLee JC, Drez D. Orthopaedic sports medicine: principles and practice. Philadelphia: WB Saunders, 1994:1041.)

Table 10.1   Muscle strength grading

GRADE	STRENGTH	DESCRIPTION
5	Normal	Full resistance
4	Good	Decreased resistance
3	Fair	Movement against gravity possible but not with resistance
2	Poor	Movement possible with gravity eliminated
1	Trace	Slight contraction felt but no movement
0	Absence	No contraction

Table 10.2   Lower extremity muscles and reflexes

SPINAL NERVE	MUSCLE	REFLEX
L1	Hip flexors	None
L2	Hip flexors	None
L3	Knee extension	None
L4	Foot dorsiflexion	Patellar
L5	Great toe extension	Posterior tibial
S1	Foot eversion	Achilles tendon

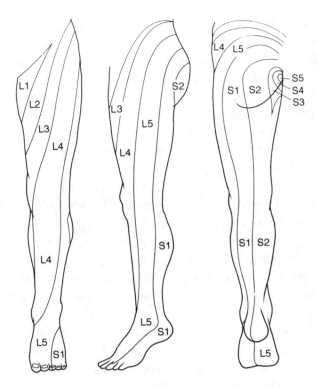

Figure 10.7 *Dermatomal distribution by spinal nerve of the lower extremity.* (Redrawn by permission from DeLee JC, Drez D. Orthopaedic sports medicine: principles and practice. Philadelphia: WB Saunders, 1994:1028.)

are then tested and reported using the standard scale 0 to 5 (Table 10.1). There is some overlap in innervation of the muscles of the lower extremity; however, most nerve roots can be isolated (Table 10.2). Next sensation should be assessed. This is best done using a small pin. The patient should be asked to close his or her eyes, and sensation should be tested in each dermatome in both lower extremities (Fig. 10.7).

Acute Thoracic and Lumbar Spine Injuries

Back pain in Western culture is an extremely common problem that affects both athletic and nonathletic population. Although the majority of back pain episodes are self-limiting, very little is known about the exact etiology of back pain. This section will discuss some suspected as well as proven causes of back pain.

Musculoligamentous Strains and Sprains

This is the most common injury of the thoracolumbar spine in athletes and leads to the greatest loss of time from practice and competition. These injuries may vary in severity from minor, with no time lost from athletic competition, to major. Muscle strains and ligamentous sprains are similar in several ways including the mechanism of injury, general pathophysiology, and treatment. It is often difficult to diagnose isolated muscular strains or ligamentous sprains in the acutely injured athlete. In fact, a significant ligamentous injury cannot occur without a concomitant muscular injury. It is, however, possible to have an isolated muscular injury without ligamentous damage. Most commonly, the injury is a combination of both a muscular strain and a ligamentous sprain.

In acute musculoligamentous injuries the history can often be diagnostic. Typically, the athlete can relate the onset of the injury to a particular event or play. There is often a history of twisting or side bending, and a sensation of tearing may be elicited. Any history of a direct blow to the thoracolumbar spine should alert the examiner to the possibility of a fracture or bony contusion. The athlete with minor injuries may continue to compete, though major injuries may leave the athlete incapacitated and unable to ambulate easily or sit comfortably. The athlete can usually easily localize the pain. It is most commonly unilateral and located in the lumbar region. However, the injury may also be bilateral and located at any point throughout the thoracolumbar spine. Typically the athlete will characterize the pain as a feeling of pulling or spasm that is significantly exacerbated by movement. As a rule the pain is isolated to the thoracolumbar region. Any pain radiating into the lower extremities should be thoroughly investigated. Because of the minor nature of the majority of these injuries, the athlete may not present for examination until 24 to 48 hours after the injury. In this situation the athlete will ordinarily give a history of continued participation initially after the injury with subsequent increasing pain and spasm.

The physical examination may vary significantly depending on the severity of the injury. Minor injuries are often not noticeable when watching the athlete walk, run, sit, or stand. However, major musculoligamentous injuries can cause severe discomfort. The athlete may have difficulty walking comfortably and often exhibits splinting on one side or the other. Sitting and standing may also be difficult and uncomfortable. Palpation typically reveals tenderness over the affected muscle group, most commonly the erector spinae complex. It is important to document the presence or absence of point tenderness over any vertebra. There may also be swelling of the musculature characteristic of intramuscular hematoma. Perhaps the most consistent finding is muscle spasm. Following an acute injury, the affected muscles can quickly enter spasm causing the muscles to feel tight. Range-of-motion test results may range from near normal to significantly limited. Often any movement exacerbates the pain. Muscle strength and sensory testing of the thoracolumbar spine is typically not necessary. However, if there is any history of pain radiating into the lower extremities, a thorough neurologic examination of the lower extremities should be performed.

The majority of acute musculoligamentous injuries in the thoracic and lumbar spine are minor and do not require evaluation by a physician. However, one must realize when examination by a physician is necessary. In general any athlete suspected of having a fracture of the thoracolumbar spine should be seen by a physician immediately and properly immobilized. This includes anyone with point bony tenderness or crepitus or a mechanism of injury that suggests the possibility of a fracture. In addition, an athlete who is significantly limited by the pain and muscle spasm should be referred to a specialist for evaluation. Most importantly, any athlete with neurologic symptoms or physical findings should be evaluated by a specialist. Any athlete originally suspected of having a minor injury who is unable to resume participation in 2 to 3 days or has significant symptoms continuing for 10 days to 2 weeks should also be referred to a specialist.

The natural courses of muscular strains and ligamentous sprains are very similar. More information regarding the response to injury and healing of these tissues can be found in Chapters 3 and 4. The goal of treatment in musculoligamentous strains and sprains of the thoracolumbar spine is the safe and speedy return of the athlete to practice and competition. The specifics of treatment are aimed at promotion and control of the normal physiology of the injury. The initial response to any strain or sprain in the thoracic and lumbar spine is inflammation and subsequent muscle spasm. Therefore the initial treatment of any athlete with an acute back injury felt to be a sprain or strain should be directed toward limiting the inflammatory response and the effects of muscle spasm. This is best accomplished by first limiting the athlete's activity for a short period of time. In minor injuries strict bed rest is not necessary, but withholding the athlete from practice for 1 to 2 days will allow the injured tissues to begin healing. In the initial 24 to 48 hours after injury, cold (ice) therapy should be used to limit inflammation and muscle spasm. The use of nonsteroidal anti-inflammatory drugs (NSAIDs) can also be helpful in limiting inflammation and controlling pain.

After the initial 48-hour period, treatment should be directed toward returning the athlete to competition as soon as possible. This entails adequate pain control and return of sufficient muscle strength and range of motion to perform the desired athletic event. Other therapeutic modalities including massage and heat therapy can be used to treat signs or symptoms of muscle spasm. The use of NSAIDs should also be continued until pain and spasm are essentially gone.

To regain the needed flexibility and strength, a program of stretching and muscle strengthening is recommended. Stretching of the thoracic and lumbar spine can be accomplished by taking the spine through its normal range of motion. All stretching should be done in a steady, consistent fashion within the limits of the patient's comfort. The movements targeted should be flexion, extension, side-to-side bending, and rotation as well as knee-to-chest stretches. Hamstring stretching should also be included in any stretching program (Fig. 10.8).

A proper strengthening program for the thoracolumbar spine should be aimed at both the paraspinal musculature and the abdominal muscles. The strengthening program for paraspinal muscles includes press-ups, hyperextensions, and pelvic tilts. Abdominal strengthening can be accomplished through abdominal crunches and straight-leg raises (Fig. 10.9). These exercises should initially be performed two to three times per day. They may be discontinued once the athlete is no longer experiencing any symptoms of pain or spasm.

Criteria for return to practice and competition vary with each individual sport. In general, the athlete is allowed to return to light practice when the pain and spasm are well controlled. It is important not to allow the athlete to overexert himself or herself in an attempt to return to competition too quickly. Flare-ups of the pain and spasm are not uncommon if activity has been resumed too quickly. When the athlete does return to practice, proper warm-up before practice and cool-down after practice are necessary. Before and after all practices heat and massage therapies can amplify the effects of stretching and strengthening exercises.

Muscular Contusion

Muscle contusions result not from a stretching injury, but from a nonpenetrating blunt injury. They also occur frequently in the

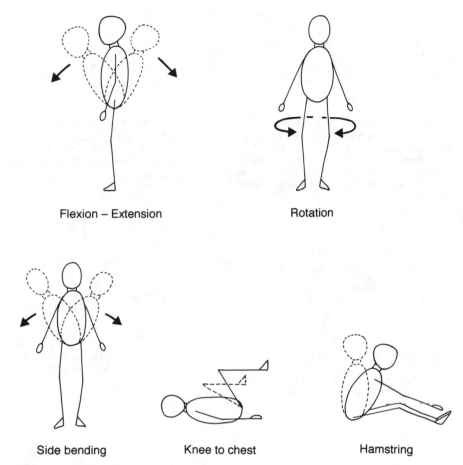

Flexion – Extension   Rotation

Side bending   Knee to chest   Hamstring

Figure 10.8 *General stretching exercises used in the treatment of low back pain.*

thoracolumbar spine of athletes and can cause significant loss of time from practice and competition.

As expected, the athlete will relate a history of suffering a direct blow to the thoracic or lumbar spine. The athlete typically is able to localize the pain exactly. The pain is similar in character to that with pulling or spasm of a muscle strain and is exacerbated by movement. The physical examination in general is also very similar to that for a muscle strain. There is tenderness on palpation over the affected muscle group, and often significant swelling and spasm. As a rule, range of motion is decreased.

The treatment of muscle contusions is identical to that of musculoligamentous strains and sprains. The initial therapy should include withholding the athlete from activity as necessary, NSAIDs,

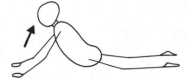

Prone press-ups: Lie on your stomach with palms near your shoulders, as if to do a standard push-up. Slowly push your shoulders up, keeping your hips on the surface and letting your back and stomach sag. Slowly lower your shoulders. Repeat 10 times.

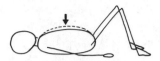

Pelvic tilt: Lie on your back with knees bent, feet flat on floor. Flatten the small of your back against the floor, without pushing down with the legs. Hold for 5 to 10 seconds.

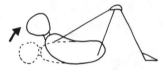

Crunch: Do the pelvic tilt and, while holding this position, slowly curl your head and shoulders off the floor. Hold briefly. Return slowly to the starting position.

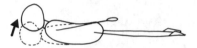

Upper back exercise: Lying on stomach with arms at sides, slowly lift head up.

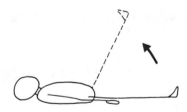

Raise one leg off ground (keeping knee straight) as high as possible then slowly lower. Repeat with opposite leg.

Figure 10.9 *General back and abdominal strengthening exercises for low back pain.* (Redrawn by permission from DeLee JC, Drez D. Orthopaedic sports medicine: principles and practice. Philadelphia: WB Saunders, 1994:1044, 1046–1047.)

and a combination of ice and heat treatments. This should be followed by massage and heat therapy, continued NSAIDs, and a stretching and strengthening program.

Return to athletic participation should be allowed gradually as the athlete's pain and spasm decrease and strength and flexibility increase. In general, most muscle contusions are minor, self-limiting injuries and do not require referral to a physician. The guidelines for referral discussed for musculoligamentous injuries also apply to muscle contusions.

Spinal Fracture and Dislocations

Fractures and dislocations of the thoracolumbar vertebrae can have severe consequences and are occasionally seen in athletics. Although an extensive discussion of these injuries is beyond the scope of this book, they are briefly discussed in order to allow recognition and appropriate handling. Any injured athlete with severe, acute back pain following obvious trauma can have a spine fracture. In particular, numbness or weakness in the lower extremities should alert the treating person to the potential of fracture or dislocation. Pain and tenderness directly over the spinous processes can be another finding. Obvious deformity of the spine and lower extremity paralysis indicate a severe injury such as a fracture or dislocation unless proven otherwise.

Fractures often involve the vertebral body, and displaced bone fragments can injure the spinal cord and nerves resulting in paralysis. These injuries are often called burst farctures. Dislocations occur when the previously described ligaments tear and allow one vertebra to separate and displace relative to another. This results in a kinking or even obliteration of the spinal canal, thereby also injuring the spinal cord and nerves. The initial approach is based on the same principles as described for neck injuries in Chapter 6. Extreme care should be taken in transporting the patient from the athletic facility to the hospital to avoid further injury to the spinal cord. Log rolling and the use of a rigid spine board are necessary to accomplish this. If a fracture or dislocation is present, then surgical correction and stabilization are often needed to allow recovery and rehabilitation.

Chronic Thoracic and Lumbar Back Pain

Many persons, including athletes of all ages, experience chronic back pain (thoracic and lumbar) on a daily basis. However, the etiologies of the pain may often be different in the athlete. For the purpose of this book we will describe chronic back pain as pain that was not preceded by a significant acute injury which could explain the symptoms and physical findings. The etiology of chronic thoracic and lumbar pain in athletes may be due to overuse, intervertebral disk disease, or structural spinal deformities.

Chronic Muscle Strain

Chronic muscle strain is thought to be a common cause of back pain. Repetitive loading of the muscles around the spine may be causing injuries on a microscopic level (see Chapter 3). Although chronic muscle strains are thought to be responsible for a large number of the cases of chronic low back pain, it remains to be proved that the initial injury actually occurred in the muscles. Other sources of pain such as the facet joint or intervertebral disks have not been ruled out.

There is typically no history of an acute back injury. The athlete will usually initially complain of a dull achy pain or tightness in the back following athletic activities. Later the pain may begin to occur during strenuous activities and finally during daily activities. Most commonly the pain is located in the lower back; however, it may be localized at any point throughout the thoracolumbar spine. There is usually no radiating pain.

Physical examination may vary depending on the severity of the symptoms and at what point one examines the patient. If the symptoms are mild, one may notice no alteration in the athlete's ability to walk, run, sit, or stand. However, if the symptoms are severe or if the examination is after a strenuous workout, the athlete may have difficulty moving in a comfortable manner. Range of motion in the thoracic and lumbar spine will most likely be decreased secondary to pain. Palpation will reveal tenderness in the muscle itself or at its insertion. There also may be appreciable muscle spasm.

In general, a chronic muscle strain is a self-limiting condition that will resolve without formal medical attention. However, if it persists for longer than 3 to 4 weeks with treatment or continues to worsen with proper treatment, the athlete should be referred to a specialist for evaluation. The treatment is centered on control of the pain and muscle spasm. The pain sometimes responds to cold therapy during a severe flare-up. NSAIDs may also be helpful. The muscle spasm can be treated with heat therapy. This should be applied before the workout to ensure that the muscles are warm and loose as well as after the workout. In addition, the athlete should be advised to stretch before and after all workouts or competitions. Lower back and abdominal strengthening exercises are also helpful. Finally, the athlete should be instructed to limit his or her activity level for a short time until the pain is under control, then gradually increase the activity to the preinjury level.

Chronic muscle strains, depending on severity, may or may not prevent the athlete from competing. Typically, the pain is not severe enough to prevent competition, although it may affect the athlete's performance. There is no risk of serious injury if the athlete continues to compete; however, the lack of rest may prolong the symptoms. If the athlete is initially unable to participate in workouts or competition because of pain, he or she may be allowed to return when the symptoms improve. This should be individualized to the athlete and the sport in which he or she is participating.

Iliac Apophysitis

Iliac apophysitis is an inflammation of the apophysis (growth plate) located on the top of each iliac wing. It occurs only in younger athletes who are not yet skeletally mature. As with chronic muscle strains, the athlete will initially complain of a dull achy pain in the lower back following athletic activities. Later the pain will begin to occur during strenuous activities and may subsequently occur during daily activities.

Physical examination will vary depending on the severity of the symptoms. Palpation will reveal tenderness along the iliac crests. There also may be appreciable muscle spasm. Range of motion in the lower back will most likely be decreased secondary to muscle spasm and pain.

As previously mentioned, iliac apophysitis comes from chronic inflammation of the apophysis (growth plate) located on top of the iliac crests of growing athletes. This is the location for many muscular attachments and is therefore subject to repetitive strain during activities. When this strain exceeds the capacity of the apophysis, the apophysis may become inflamed. This inflammatory reaction causes pain and tenderness in the area and can also lead to muscle spasm. In general iliac apophysitis is a self-limiting condition that will often resolve without formal medical attention. The symptomatic treatment is essentially the same as that for a chronic muscle strain because the etiology and symptoms are very similar.

Lumbar Interspinous Bursitis

Lumbar interspinous bursitis (kissing spines) is caused by irritation and inflammation of the bursa between the spinous processes of the lumbar vertebrae. As with other etiologies of chronic back pain, its onset is often slow and there is typically no history of an acute injury. The pain is dull in nature and located in the lumbar region. The athlete will often report that the pain is exacerbated by hyperextension of the lumbar spine and decreases with flexion. There is usually no radiation of the pain.

Physical examination may reveal no alteration in walking, running, sitting, or standing. Palpation will reveal tenderness between the two spinous processes involved, the most common level being L4 and L5. Often there is also spasm of the surrounding musculature. Range of motion will be limited secondary to pain and spasm. This is most often noted in extension, which typically causes worsening of the pain.

The etiology of this condition is related to repetitive rubbing of one spinous process on another from hyperextension of the lumbar spine. Because of its mechanism, this condition is common in gymnasts. The repetitive contact between the two spinous processes leads to irritation and inflammation of the bursae.

Treatment is aimed toward relief of the bursitis. This is accomplished through limiting activities for a short period of time. The use of ice or NSAIDs may also be helpful. The athlete rarely misses a significant amount of time secondary to this condition. Pain is the only factor limiting activities, and the athlete may be allowed to return to activities when the pain is controlled.

Spondylolysis and Spondylolisthesis

Spondylolysis and spondylolisthesis are not uncommon causes of back pain in athletes. Spondylolysis refers to a defect in the pars interarticularis of the posterior elements of the lumbar spine, and spondylolisthesis refers to the anterior displacement of one vertebra on another secondary to this defect (Fig. 10.10).

The presentation of spondylolysis and spondylolisthesis can vary from a lack of symptoms to severe pain. The pain is typically nondescript, although the back pain is somewhat chronic in nature. There is usually no history of trauma. The pain is usually relieved by rest. Occasionally, there may be pain radiating down both legs.

On physical examination, findings in spondylolysis and spondy-

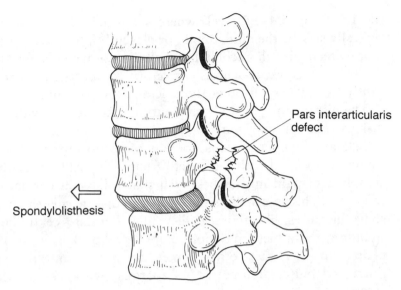

Figure 10.10 *A pars interarticularis defect and associated spondylolisthesis.*

lolisthesis may be limited to localized tenderness on palpation in the affected area of the lumbar spine. In the presence of spondylolisthesis, there may also be a palpable step off at the level of the slip. There is also loss of lumbar range of motion. Examination of the lower extremities may reveal hamstring tightness, but there are rarely any neurologic findings.

There are several causes of spondylolysis and spondylolisthesis, and a full discussion of these is beyond the scope of this chapter. However, the most common etiology in athletes is a stress fracture. The theorized cause of a stress fracture in the pars interarticularis is repetitive hyperextension of the lumbar spine. This motion causes repetitive stress concentrated in the pars interarticularis, which initially leads to a stress reaction. With continued hyperextension, a true stress fracture may develop. Any athlete suspected of having spondylolysis or spondylolisthesis should be referred to a specialist for evaluation and treatment. Treatment and guidelines for returning to athletic participation should also be determined by a specialist.

Thoracic and Lumbar Disk Disease

Thoracic and lumbar disk degeneration and herniation are, in general, uncommon in the athlete. The most common situation for disk disease in the athlete would be the older athlete with a lumbar disk. When they do occur, some 95% of lumbar disk herniations occur at the L5–S1 or L4–L5 level, whereas thoracic disk herniations are typically seen at the ninth, tenth, or eleventh interspaces. It is important to recognize thoracolumbar disk disease when it does occur, as the treatment and prognosis for return to sports may vary significantly from those for other thoracic and lumbar injuries.

The history and physical examination of an athlete with a thoracic disk herniation may vary significantly. As compared with acute muscle and ligament strains, there is often no history of significant trauma associated with the onset of pain. Typically, the athlete will complain of pain in the chest wall that follows a dermatomal distribution. This is usually seen when the disk herniates laterally. In some instances, the thoracic disk may herniate centrally. In this situation, the athlete may not complain of back pain at all. Complaints in this case often center on the feeling of spasticity (increased muscular tone) or paraparesis (weakness) of the lower extremities.

The physical examination in an athlete with a thoracic disk herniation can also have variable results. Inspection may reveal no abnormality. Palpation may localize tenderness in the area of the disk herniation. The range of motion of the thoracic spine is likely to be decreased secondary to pain. With lateral thoracic disk herniations, the physical examination may reveal paresthesias (abnormal sensation) in the chest wall in a dermatomal distribution. With central disk herniations, physical examination may reveal increased reflexes in the lower extremities or spastic paraparesis. It should be emphasized that thoracic disk herniations are rare. Any athlete suspected of having a thoracic disk herniation should be referred to a specialist for further evaluation and possible surgical treatment.

Evaluation of the athlete with a suspected lumbar disk degeneration or herniation should again begin with the history. The pain that is associated with disk degeneration is often very similar to a pain of muscular origin. It can be located in the midline or paraspinal region. As with thoracic disk disease, there is often no history of injury or only minor injury before the onset of pain. The pain may be exacerbated by activities.

The pain with a lumbar disk herniation can often be variable as well. The athlete may complain of mainly low back and buttock pain. However, if there is radiating leg pain (sciatica) as well as back pain, a disk herniation should be suspected. The herniated disk material (Fig. 10.11) will compress and irritate the spinal nerve that exits the

Herniated disk

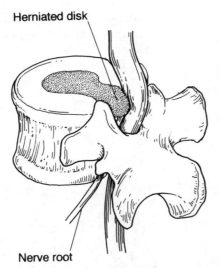

Nerve root

Figure 10.11 *A herniated interverte-bral disk with compression of the nerve root.*

spinal canal. This causes pain down the posterior aspect of the leg. If the compression is more severe, permanent numbness and weakness in the leg can occur.

The physical examination of the athlete will vary with disk degeneration or herniation. In both situations, there may be some mild tenderness to palpation over the area of disk disease. On inspection, one may also notice some flattening of the lumbar contour secondary to muscle spasm. Range of motion of the lumbar spine is often limited in both conditions secondary to muscle spasm.

The key in differentiating between disk degeneration and herniation is the physical examination of the lower extremities. A thorough neurologic evaluation of the lower extremities to include muscle strength testing, sensory testing, flexes, and the presence or absence of tension signs must be documented. The patient should be asked to toe walk and heel walk. The specific muscle groups to be tested should include the hip flexors, knee extensors, foot dorsiflexors and everters, great toe extensor, and foot plantar flexors. A sensory examination of the lower extremities should be performed by testing the patient's ability to feel pin pricks throughout the dermatomes of the lower extremities. Reflexes including knee jerk, ankle jerk, and posterior tibialis should be tested. Sciatic nerve tension signs should be tested, as they are very sensitive indicators of nerve root compression. The best sciatic nerve tension test is the straight-leg raise. This should be performed with the patient lying supine on the table. The

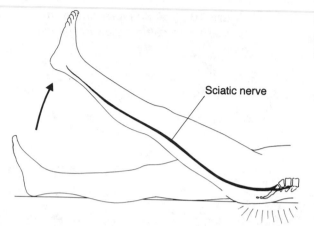

Figure 10.12 *Straight-leg-raising test to elicit nerve root pain.*

Sciatic nerve

leg is raised with the knee fully extended. To be positive, the test should reproduce the patient's leg pain (Fig. 10.12). It is not considered positive if only back pain is produced.

An initial bout of back pain with sciatica can often be managed by a short period of rest, analgesics, and physical modalities. Most disk herniations will gradually resolve without long-term risks. In chronic cases or in the presence of neurologic deficits such as muscle weakness or bowel or bladder problems, further studies may be needed. A magnetic resonance imaging (MRI) scan or myelogram can determine the exact pathology and aid in the planning of surgery for these cases.

Scoliosis and Kyphosis

Chronic deformities of the spine are not uncommon and generally do not prevent the affected person from active sports participation. Both scoliosis and kyphosis are often asymptomatic. Chronic back pain in a young athlete with a spinal deformity should prompt a search for another underlying cause of the pain and possibly the deformity.

Scoliosis is an abnormal lateral curvature of the spine. When viewed from behind the individual with scoliosis may have an obvious lateral deformity of the spine. This deformity is often better seen when the athlete is asked to bend forward and touch his or her toes. In this position, the rib hump that is characteristic of scoliosis is typically prominent. Kyphosis is characterized as excessive flexion of the thoracic spine. As a rule, a kyphotic deformity is easily recognized, especially when the patient is viewed from the side. Both deformities should be evaluated by a specialist to determine whether any treatment is warranted. If the condition is severe enough to warrant treatment, both bracing and surgery are used. In both scoliosis and kyphosis the normal range of motion of the thoracic and lumbar spine is altered.

Differential Diagnosis of Back Pain

Acute Pain

- ✘ Acute muscular strain
- ✘ Muscular contusion
- ✘ Vertebral fracture or dislocation
- ✘ Acute flare-up of a chronic condition (e.g., chronic strain or herniated disk)

Chronic Pain

- ✘ Chronic muscular strain
- ✘ Iliac apophysitis
- ✘ Lumbar interspinous bursitis
- ✘ Spondylolysis and spondylolisthesis
- ✘ Thoracic and lumbar disk disease

Suggested Readings

American Academy of Orthopaedic Surgeons. Athletic training and sports medicine. 2nd ed. Park Ridge, IL: American Academy of Orthopaedic Surgeons, 1991.

Chilton MD, Nisenfeld FG. Nonoperative treatment of low back injury in athletes. Clin Sports Med 1993;12(3):547–555.

Delee JC, Drez D Jr, eds. Orthopaedic sports medicine: principles and practice, vol. 2. Philadelphia: WB Saunders, 1994:1018–1062.

Grana WA, Kalenak A, eds. Clinical sports medicine. Philadelphia: WB Saunders, 1991:402–412.

Harvey J, Tanner S. Low back pain in young athletes. A practical approach. Sports Med 1991;12(6):394–406.

Keene JS, Drummond DS. Mechanical back pain in the athlete. Compr Ther 1985;11(1):7–14.

CHAPTER 11

Hip, Pelvis, and Thigh Injuries

Bryan W. Smith and O. E. Tillman

The hip, pelvis, and thigh area contains many powerful muscles that contribute to acceleration and deceleration in virtually all athletic activities. The envelope of large muscles around the bones and joints in this area also provides excellent shock absorption during impact and falls. Therefore bone and joint injuries are relatively uncommon in the hip, pelvis, and thigh area. However, soft tissue injuries and in particular muscle injuries make up the majority of the injuries in this area. This chapter will discuss the most common soft tissue injuries in both the hip and pelvis as well as the thigh area.

Hip and Pelvis

When compared with injuries to the shoulder, knee, and ankle, athletic injuries to the hip and pelvis are relatively uncommon. However, proper function of this area of the body is essential for successful performance in sports. In running, more than four times one's body weight is transmitted across the hip joint. Injuries to the hip and pelvis can be difficult to diagnose and manage. Some of the injuries involve the bony architecture and will not be discussed in detail. Soft tissue injuries are more frequent. They include acute injuries such as contusions and muscle strains, as well as chronic injuries such as tendinitis and bursitis.

The anatomy of the hip and pelvis is complex. The pelvis can be seen as a bony ring that forms a joint with the sacrum and remaining spine through the sacroiliac joints posteriorly (Fig. 11.1). The ring

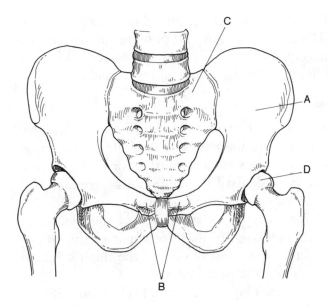

Figure 11.1 *Bony structures of the hip and pelvis: the ilium (A), the pubis (B), the sacrum (C), and the hip joint (D).*

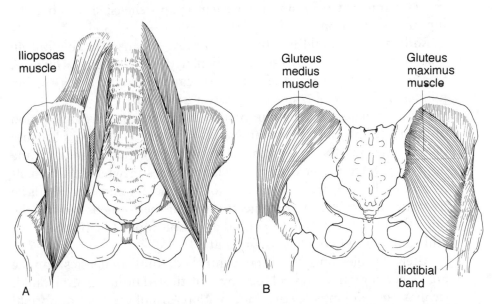

Figure 11.2 *Major muscle of the anterior (A) and posterior (B) hip and pelvis.*

consists of the sacrum, the ilium and its iliac wings, the ischium, and the pubic rami. The hip joint consists of a deep socket or acetabulum and a perfectly round femoral head. Several muscles are involved in hip motion (Fig. 11.2). Primary hip flexors are the iliopsoas, rectus femoris, and sartorius. Extension utilizes the gluteus maximus and hamstring muscles. The gluteus medius and minimus along with the tensor fascia lata are responsible for hip abduction. The adductors, brevis, magnus, and longus, primarily control hip adduction.

Hip and Pelvic Contusions

A hip pointer refers to a contusion to the iliac crest. Anyone who has suffered this injury can attest to the pain and disability it can cause. It usually occurs in contact sports such as football or hockey. However, falls to the floor in basketball or volleyball or contact with equipment in gymnastics can result in hip pointers.

Numerous muscles have origins or insertions at the iliac crest, which explains the extreme disability that accompanies this injury. Rotation or bending of the trunk and flexion of the thigh are quite painful as the muscles pull on the contused area.

Usually these contusions are easy to diagnose. Ecchymosis may not be visible. However, the patient may have an abrasion. Palpation causes significant pain, and the patient is apprehensive to move the hip in any direction.

Radiographs should be obtained in most instances to rule out an iliac crest fracture or avulsion, particularly in the young athlete. A tear of the muscle near the iliac crest can be confused with a hip pointer. A history of contact suggests a hip pointer.

Initial management of a hip pointer includes ice and compression of the area. This must be maintained for as long as 48 hours because of the tendency for slow bleeding to occur overnight, making the disability worse the next day. In selected cases in which a fluctuant mass can be palpated, aspiration of the hematoma under sterile technique and corticosteroid injection may be performed. Most of the time, the hematoma is not localized and aspiration is ineffective. The athlete may need crutches to ambulate.

After the bleeding has been controlled, oral analgesics can be prescribed for pain. Physical therapy is instituted utilizing ultrasound, ice massage, and muscle stretching, with return of the joint to normal range of motion being the goal.

Return to activity is variable but usually is in 1 to 3 weeks. A potential complication is myositis ossificans (see the section below on quadriceps contusion). Protective padding to prevent reinjury is important. It is just as important to make sure that the uniform padding fits properly and has not been altered. This can prevent these injuries from ever occurring.

Bursitis Around the Hip and Pelvis

There are at least 13 permanent bursae around the hip and pelvis, localized between tendons and muscles and over bony prominences. Bursitis (inflammation of the bursa) can occur in anyone, but is especially bothersome in the athlete. Proper diagnosis and treatment are essential in helping the athlete return to full sports participation. This section will outline the clinical features and management of both traumatic and inflammatory hip bursitis in athletes.

Traumatic Bursitis

Traumatic or hemorrhagic bursitis is most commonly caused by a direct trauma or blow to the bursae, as when an athlete's hip strikes a hard playing surface. This injury can also be caused indirectly through bleeding from an adjacent muscle or tendon strain. On physical examination, tenderness, soft tissue swelling, and fluctuation may be noted. Proper treatment is essential to help prevent long-term disability. An acute hemorrhagic bursitis may be evacuated using an 18- or 19-gauge needle under sterile conditions. An elastic wrap bandage may then be applied for compression. If this condition is not treated adequately, the blood will coagulate, and eventually fibrinous adhesive tissue and fibrin bodies will form in the bursa. These adhesions will produce a chronic inflammatory bursitis with recurrent problems. When this happens, surgical excision of the bursa may be required. Traumatic bursitis can often be prevented by adequate protective padding, such as that used by goalkeepers in field hockey or soccer.

Inflammatory Bursitis

Three bursa around the hip are most commonly involved in inflammatory reactions in athletes: the trochanteric, psoas (or iliopectineal), and ischial (Fig. 11.3). These injuries are most frequently the result of friction caused by repetitive movements of a muscle or tendon against a bursa. The onset of pain is usually gradual but progresses to become proportional to activity.

Trochanteric Bursitis: Trochanteric bursitis usually manifests as a burning or deep aching sensation over or just behind the tip of the greater trochanter. The pain is made worse with activity and may be referred down the lateral aspect of the thigh with certain movements of the hip. On examination tenderness is localized over the greater

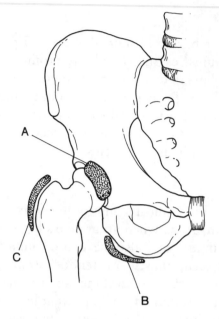

Figure 11.3 *Major bursae around the hip and pelvis: psoas bursa (A), the ischial bursa (B), and the trochanteric bursa (C).*

trochanter, and pain is reproduced with external rotation of the hip and with adduction of the leg.

This condition is frequently seen in runners and ballet dancers. In runners who train on outdoor surfaces, symptoms are usually noted on the "down-side" leg (related to the camber of the road), which produces a functional leg-length discrepancy. In runners whose feet cross the midline, their abnormal mechanics increase the adduction angle and increase friction between the trochanter and overlying iliotibial band. Either mechanism will increase friction between the iliotibial tract and the greater trochanter and can irritate the bursa. Bursitis development in dancers is thought to be related to a combination of repetitive, full-range hip work, one-legged balance maneuvers, and imbalanced flexibility with a tight iliotibial band. Therefore avoidance of training errors and adequate flexibility appear to be the key preventive measures.

Initial treatment includes relative rest, icing, stretching exercises (with special emphasis on the iliotibial band), and nonsteroidal anti-inflammatory drugs. If symptoms persist, a series of local injections with local anesthetic and corticosteroids may be of benefit. Orthotics are also useful on occasion. In resistant cases, surgical excision of the inflamed bursa and a small portion of the iliotibial band is considered.

Psoas Bursitis: The psoas bursa is the largest synovial bursa in the body and communicates with the hip joint in about 15% of adults. It is located anterior to the hip joint and dorsal to the iliopsoas tendon. Athletes usually complain of disabling midgroin pain, made worse with activity, which may radiate into the medial thigh. A characteristic antalgic gait with the hip held in mild flexion and external rotation may also be noted. The midgroin will be exquisitely tender on examination, and pain may be reproduced with full internal and external hip rotation and resisted hip flexion.

Treatment includes relative rest, nonsteroidal medication, electrical stimulation, and ultrasound therapy. If symptoms persist, local injection with corticosteroids and local anesthetic agents may help. As symptoms improve, gentle hip flexion exercises are begun, with a slow progression of activities as the athlete's pain allows.

Ischial Bursitis: Ischial bursitis is usually caused by a direct fall onto the buttocks. However, there is often a history of prolonged sitting, especially with the legs crossed or on a hard surface, which has led some to refer to this condition as "benchwarmer's bursitis."

Examination reveals tenderness over the ischial bursa. This condition must be differentiated from other peri-ischial pathology including avulsion of the hamstrings, apophysitis in adolescents, osteomyelitis, and neoplastic disorders.

Treatment recommendations follow the same program as outlined for the other bursae. In addition, the use of a donut-shaped pillow during sitting can decrease the friction and thereby the symptoms of bursitis. The athlete usually responds to conservative measures, and surgical intervention is rarely required.

Muscle Strains

Injuries or strain to the muscle-tendon unit usually involve a partial or complete tear of the muscle tissue. They often occur during a forceful lengthening contraction of the affected muscle. Other general information on the biomechanics, pathology, and injury response can be found in Chapters 2, 3, and 4. These injuries are not uncommon around the hip and pelvis because of the large number of muscles in this area. The most common strains will be discussed in this section.

Hip Flexor Strains

Iliopsoas strains result from forceful attempts to flex the hip while the thigh is fixed or pushed in extension. The injury usually occurs near the musculotendinous junction near the insertion at the lesser trochanter. Avulsion fracture at the lesser trochanter can occur in adolescents but is unusual and seldom requires surgical management. The most common sports for these injuries are gymnastics, track (hurdling), and swimming. Rectus femoris and sartorius muscle injuries are discussed below in the thigh section of this chapter.

Symptoms consist of deep groin pain, usually difficult to localize but exacerbated by hip flexion. The pain may extend into the lower abdomen. Weight bearing may be difficult. The patient may also complain of a snapping sensation. This can be due to damage to the soft tissue surrounding the tendon or to inflammation of the tendon sheath itself.

On physical examination, one can palpate tenderness in the groin lateral to the neurovascular bundle. Pain can be elicited by stretching the tendon by extending and internally rotating the hip. Another motion that can cause a snapping sensation or pain is to duplicate the trail leg motion of a hurdler. The hip flexor strength is reduced and may be painful against resistance.

Radiographs of the hip should be negative unless an avulsion is present. Young children and early adolescents should always have x-rays taken to rule out hip disorders such as Legg-Perthes disease or slipped capital femoral epiphysis.

Treatment consists of relative rest from aggravating activities, non-steroidal anti-inflammatory drugs, and physical therapy. Range-of-motion and strengthening activities are encouraged. This allows a progressive return to activity. In some recalcitrant cases, steroid injections or surgical management or both can be required.

Hip Extensor Strains

In terms of hip extension, the gluteus maximus is the primary functioning muscle. This large muscle has a broad origin and a number of insertions including the iliotibial tract and the proximal femur. The muscle is seldom injured. Most injuries involve the weaker hip extensors, being the hamstrings, piriformis, and gluteus medius. Strains to these muscles will be discussed in more detail.

Hip Abductor Strains

Gluteus medius strains with associated tendinitis at the greater trochanteric insertion are occasionally seen. Running, swimming, football, and hockey are the sports that have the greatest number of such injuries. Although the mechanism of injury is uncertain, it is possibly a seesaw pelvic tilt action that leads to fatigue in the muscle and subsequent injury.

On physical examination one can usually palpate tenderness proximal to the greater trochanter. There is also pain on resisted hip abduction. Varus alignment and leg-length discrepancy are frequently found. Passive range of motion is usually not affected. This is in contrast to trochanteric bursitis, which will be tender with range-of-motion testing. A small percentage of patients may have both entities.

In young adolescents, there is a possibility of an avulsion of the gluteus medius at the greater trochanteric insertion. This would result in severe pain and disability. X-rays should always be obtained when there is a question of an avulsion. This injury usually requires orthopedic attention unless there is only a minimal degree of separation. In these cases, hip spica fixation or protected weight bearing is needed.

Treatment of gluteal strains requires relative rest, physical therapy, and nonsteroidal anti-inflammatory medications. Corticosteroid injection may benefit concomitant bursitis. Altering the surfaces the athlete runs on may prevent future episodes. Significant alignment problems need to be corrected.

Hip Adductor Strains

Numerous muscles are invovled in hip adduction. Most injuries in sports involve the adductor longus. Mechanisms such as quick bursts of adduction and abduction of the leg, as seen in passing and shooting a soccer ball, can result in injury. Repetitive movements, such as those found in breaststroking, can cause fatigue and subsequent injury. Occasionally, the injury results from a sudden abduction from slipping on a wet surface. Other than soccer and swimming, adductor strains are occasionally seen in skating, football, rugby, hockey, and equestrian sports.

Tendon avulsions from the origin at the inferior pubic ramus rarely occur. Usually the muscle strain is located at the musculotendinous junction in the upper third of the muscle. Complete ruptures of the muscle are found in the distal third of the muscle near the femoral insetion.

Symptoms vary depending on whether the injury is acute or chronic. Acute injury results in sharp groin pain that may radiate into the thigh. The athlete's ability to play will be limited depending on the extent of the strain. Hemorrhage and swelling may be difficult to appreciate except in severe injuries. With complete tears (grade III), a soft tissue thigh mass may be seen and palpated. Pain may be less than expected.

The chronic strain is characterized by vague and variable symptoms. Stiffness with inactivity that decreases with easy exercise is commonly found. However, intense activity results in pain. These symptoms often have an insidious onset.

On physical examination a soft tissue mass, edema, or ecchymoses may be found. Tenderness may be elicited with direct palpation, and pain may be induced with either passive abduction or resisted adduction of the hip. Radiographs may reveal dystrophic calcification at the adductor origin in chronic cases.

Treatment initially consists of rest, ice, and compression if possible. Crutches may be necessary, but early range-of-motion exercise is encouraged after the first 24 hours. Nonsteroidal anti-inflammatory medication may be started at this time to augment a progressive physical therapy program. To maintain general conditioning, cycling and freestyle or backstroke swimming is encouraged early. Surgery is rarely indicated even in grade III strains.

Return to activity can be considered when adductor strength is at least 80% of the quadriceps strength and full range of motion is restored. This may take as many as 12 weeks in chronic cases. Adductor strains have a tendency to recur if activities are resumed prematurely.

Piriformis Syndrome

Piriformis syndrome is a constellation of symptoms with posterior pelvic pain and radiation into the leg. It has been questioned as a true entity, but some athletes with these symptoms seem to fit the diagnosis and respond to the recommended treatment. However, there is no absolute proof that this condition truly exists, and often the diagnosis is made by exclusion of others.

The piriformis muscle originates on the anterior sacrum and inserts on the greater trochanter. The sciatic nerve usually travels posterior to the piriformis, but in approximately 15% of individuals, the nerve may travel through the muscle or superiorly (Fig. 11.4). The primary action of the piriformis is to externally rotate the hip. Piriformis syndrome occurs when the sciatic nerve becomes irritated via trauma to the piriformis or when muscle spasm affects the nerve. Although the syndrome is more common in women, there does not appear to be a predominance in any particular sport.

In most patients, a history of hip trauma can be obtained. Other historical clues are pain with prolonged sitting, difficulty climbing stairs, and a recent increase in activity. There is no bowel or bladder

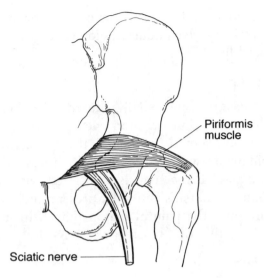

Figure 11.4 *Most common anatomic relation between piriformis muscle and sciatic nerve.*

Piriformis muscle

Sciatic nerve

dysfunction. The patient complains of deep midbuttock pain with possible sciatic radiation down the posterior thigh.

On physical examination one can demonstrate point tenderness in the sciatic notch. A rectal or vaginal examination will demonstrate piriformis tenderness proximal to the ischial spine. Lumbar range of motion is usually normal and without pain. Weakness of the hip on abduction and external rotation is found. Pain from forced internal rotation of the extended thigh (Freiberg's test) can be demonstrated. Hamstring tightness may be seen. Straight-leg raising sign or any other distal neurologic signs are not found (see Chapter 10).

There are no specific laboratory tests to confirm piriformis syndrome. Many other disorders such as lumbar disk disease, sacroiliitis, or lumbar facet syndrome can be confused with piriformis syndrome and should be considered in the differential diagnosis. Appropriate radiographic and laboratory studies may be required.

Treatment for piriformis syndrome is usually conservative by concentrating on stretching not only the piriformis but also the hamstrings and the hip extensors. Ultrasound, nonsteroidal anti-inflammatory medications, and local anesthetic injections can be used as needed. Rarely, surgical release is required.

Snapping Hip

The snapping or clicking hip is a frequent complaint among athletes, but it is associated with pain in fewer than one third of the cases. Snapping hips can be categorized as internal (medial) or external (lateral). Contributing factors to this phenomenon include muscle imbalance, improper training techniques, biomechanical mal-alignment, and imbalanced flexibility.

External or Lateral Snapping Hip

External snapping hip sensations are usually caused by either the iliotibial band or the gluteus maximus tendon over the greater tro-chanter. Physical examination should distinguish the source of the snap. The lateral snapping can usually be clearly felt through direct palpation during the snapping. If the snap is associated with pain, then an associated trochanteric bursitis is usually present and a local injection of 1% lidocaine into the painful region may help in the diagnosis. Treatment follows that of a trochanteric bursitis.

Internal or Medial Snapping Hip

The most common cause of a snapping hip is the suction phenomenon in the joint itself. Athletes may experience this painless clicking sensa-tion during sit-ups or with hip flexion movements. This condition requires no treatment.

Internal snapping may also be caused by the iliofemoral ligament over the femoral head or by the iliopsoas tendon over the lesser trochanter or iliopectineal eminence. This deep snapping sensation is usually more intense and can be demonstrated by specialized radio-graphic dye techniques. Surgical lengthening of the iliopsoas tendon has been successful in treating this condition. Less common, but more serious causes of internal hip snapping include various intra-articular abnormalities such as synovial chondromatosis, loose bodies, osteo-chondritis dessicans, labral tear, and subluxation. These conditions should be investigated with plain films, computed tomography, or arthrograms and may require surgical intervention.

Fractures

Acute fractures to the pelvis or hip require enormous forces and therefore are relatively uncommon in athletes. Pelvic fractures are notorious for their complications due to internal bleeding and injury to urologic structures. They require immediate transfer of the patient to a major trauma center. Hip fractures are common in elderly patients but fortunately are not frequent in young athletes. Because of their risk of displacement and damage to the blood supply of the femoral head, they often require surgical treatment.

More common than acute fractures are chronic stress fractures in the hip. They are seen most often in long distance runners and can occur in the pubic ramus as well as the femoral neck. The femoral neck fracture requires quick diagnosis and potential surgical treatment because of the risk of converting the stress fracture to a complete, acute fracture. Unrelenting groin pain with running should alert the physician, and appropriate referral is needed.

Thigh

Similar to the pelvis, the thigh has a substantial muscluar envelope. The quadriceps and hamstring muscles make up the majority of thigh muscles (Fig. 11.5). Both acute and chronic injuries are seen in the thigh. Acute soft tissue injuries to the thigh can be confined to two major categories, contusions and muscle strains. These injuries are so common that many are inadequately managed. The majority are preventable by recognizing the risk factors involved with the development of these injuries. Chronic injuries include myositis ossificans, meralgia paresthetica, and iliotibial band friction syndrome. The latter will be discussed in Chapter 12 on knee injuries. When evaluating thigh pain, the examiner should always keep in mind that hip pathology can give referred pain in the thigh area. A thorough hip examination is therefore mandatory. Commonly overlooked hip pathology includes femoral neck stress fractures in adults and Legg-Perthes disease or slipped capital femoral epiphysis in children.

Quadriceps Contusion

The most common contusion of significance in athletes is that of the quadriceps contusion or charley horse. This injury results from blunt trauma to the poorly padded or nonprotected anterior or anterolateral aspect of the thigh. In sports such as rugby, soccer, football, and hockey, injuries to the quadriceps are frequent, but the majority are insignificant and do not require medical attention.

Any injury that limits the athlete's ability to participate should be regarded as significant. Prompt diagnosis and management can minimize the time lost from practice and competition. This may reduce complications such as myositis ossificans and compartment syndrome. The goals of prompt treatment are to minimize bleeding and edema, prevent further injury, protect range of motion, and promote healing. An immediate aggressive management plan can allow some

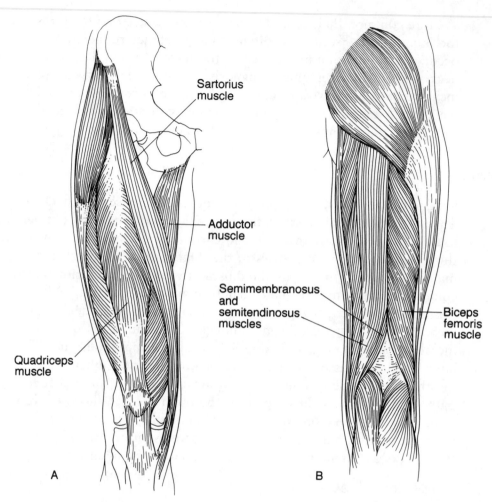

Figure 11.5 *Major muscles of the anterior (A) and posterior (B) thigh.*

athletes whose contusion has forced them from competition to return to activity in an average of 3 to 4 days. This involves immediate flexion of the knee to 120° and maintenance with an elastic wrap, which serves as an effective tamponade to control bleeding. Icing is used concomitantly. Physical therapy is started the next day, and when the athlete has regained strength and flexion without pain, return to play is allowed with protective padding. Deep massage should be avoided as it may result in further hemorrhage.

The most common complication from quadriceps contusion is myositis ossificans, which is demonstrable by x-ray 2 to 6 weeks after injury (Fig. 11.6). Usually associated with more severe injury or

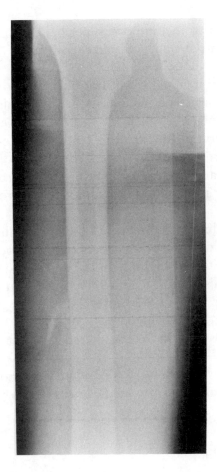

Figure 11.6 *X-ray of myositis ossificans in the thigh following blunt soft tissue trauma.*

recurrent injuries, symptoms are increased pain with activity, decreased range of motion, and a quadriceps mass. This must be differentiated from osteogenic sarcoma. Radiographic appearance, alkaline phosphatase measurement, and occasionally biopsy may be required to ensure the diagnosis.

Physical activity should be restricted, anti-inflammatory medications prescribed, and a slow progression of physical therapy followed as the bone mass is resorbed or matures. Surgical management for myositis ossificans is seldom required and should be avoided until the mass matures to avoid recurrence. This usually takes a minimum of 6 months.

Meralgia Paresthetica

The lateral femoral cutaneous nerve is a sensory nerve that supplies the anterolateral portion of the thigh down to the knee. Its peripheral entry from the pelvis is adjacent to the anterior superior iliac spine, and this nerve can run adjacent to or tunnel within the sartorius (Fig. 11.7).

The nerve can be contused or irritated from direct trauma to the area of the anterior superior iliac spine. Gymnasts are particularly vulnerable when they hit the lower parallel bar incorrectly. Other mechanisms of injury are avulsion of the sartorius from the anterior superior iliac spine and direct pressure to the nerve. The latter occurs most often in pregnancy but can develop as an overuse syndrome from wearing clothes that are too tight, for example, in aerobic dancers.

The athlete complains of tingling or numbness in the anterolateral area of the thigh. A neurologic examination is necessary, and occasionally Tinel's sign may be elicited by tapping on the anterior superior iliac spine. A positive Tinel's sign is signified by tingling in the lateral thigh while the examiner taps on the nerve. The history and physical examination should be adequate for diagnosis, but intrapelvic and spinal pathology need to be considered in questionable cases.

Treatment involves removal of the pressure source, activity modification, and nonsteroidal anti-inflammatory medications. Return of

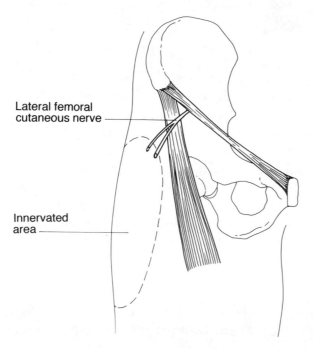

Lateral femoral
cutaneous nerve

Innervated
area

Figure 11.7 *Course and distribution of the lateral femoral cutaneous nerve.*

normal sensation usually takes a few weeks. Steroid injection may be required in persistent cases. Rarely, surgical release of the nerve appears to be the only method of obtaining complete relief.

Muscle Strains

Hamstring, quadriceps, and adductor muscles are the major groups of thigh muscles. For athletes and nonathletes, strains of these muscles are a common occurrence and reoccurrence. Adductor strains are discussed above in the secton on hip and pelvis.

Hamstring Strains

The hamstring muscles are formed in the posterior aspect of the thigh. This group is composed of the biceps femoris laterally and the semitendinosus and semimembranosus medially (see Fig. 11.5). This group of muscles functions as both hip extensors and knee flexors along with rotating the leg. A primary role of the hamstring muscles is to decelerate the leg.

Although the hamstring muscles are the most common muscles in the thigh to be strained, the exact mechanism of injury is unknown. One theory is simultaneous contraction of the quadriceps and the biceps femoris. With the hamstring muscles having only two thirds the strength of the quadriceps, it is possible that the hamstrings are overpowered.

As in most strains, the most common site of injury is the musculotendinous junction. However, in youngsters with open apophyses, avulsion fracture can be more common and must always be considered. The origin of the hamstrings is the ischial tuberosity.

The degree of injury dictates the symptoms experienced. First degree (grade I) strains, consisting of microtears in the muscle, are tender at the site of injury with activity or direct palpation. No defect in the muscle can be palpated, and minimal soft tissue edema is evident. More of the soreness may be due to muscle spasm than to muscle tearing.

A second degree (grade II) strain results from partial tearing of the muscle fibers. Pain, ecchymosis, and increased soft tissue edema are found. A muscle defect may be palpable depending on the degree of the tear. There is increased muscle spasm to protect the injury, and this is evidenced by a loss of knee extension. Functional testing of the muscle demonstrates weakness.

A third degree (grade III) strain indicates a complete muscle tear. Severe pain, disability, and gross ecchymoses are evident. A palpable defect in the muscle can be found on physical examination. However, this defect may be obscured by hematoma if the injury is evaluated several hours after it occurs.

Avulsion fracture should be suspected if the ischial tuberosity is tender when palpated. In this situation, x-rays should be obtained, and if the degree of displacement is more than 8 mm, the likelihood of bone healing is poor. Orthopedic referral should be made.

The initial management for any degree of hamstring strain involves rest, ice, compression, and elevation (RICE) therapy for 24 to 72 hours depending on the extent of the injury. Nonsteroidal anti-inflammatory medications, physical therapy, and other modalities are then employed to restore active range of motion. Return to activity is dictated by the restoration of full range of motion and at least 80% to 85% of strength.

Inadequate rehabilitation increases the risk of reinjury. The more reinjury, the more scarring occurs, and the greater the chance of reinjury. A program of warm-up and stretching should be stressed to the athlete to minimize reinjury. Hamstring taping or knee bracing to prevent hyperextension may protect the muscle when the athlete returns to activity.

Quadriceps Strain

Quadriceps strains are uncommon relative to hamstring strains. They usually result from a violent, forceful contraction of the muscles as in kicking a ball. Other possible mechanisms are unexpected, sudden muscle accelerations or decelerations as in sprinting. The muscle that is usually affected is the rectus femoris owing to its function as a two-joint muscle. Occasionally, the sartorius can be strained in soccer and football kickers.

Pain, spasm, and disability are common symptoms depending on the degree and location of the strain. Peripheral tears cause lesser symptoms than deep muscle tears. On clinical examination point tenderness is evident and palpable with strains of grade II and above. Muscle defect may be found prior to hematoma formation. Grade III strains usually result in a deformity of the anterior thigh. Edema and ecchymoses are seen locally but may be found in the distal extremity owing to gravity. Significant strains result in limited active knee flexion, with pain and spasm restricting motion.

Tendon ruptures at the superior pole of the patella should alert the examiner to the possibility of steroid use or illnesses such as collagen vascular disease or chronic inflammatory diseases. These injuries usually require surgical management. In young athletes, avulsion injuries of the quadriceps result in injury to the anterior superior iliac spine (sartorius) or to the anterior inferior iliac spine (rectus femoris). Palpation of these muscle origins should always be performed and x-rays obtained in cases of suspected injury.

Sartorius avulsions tend to displace inferiorly and entrap the lateral femoral cutaneous nerve. This results in sensation changes of numbness or tingling over the anteromedial area of the thigh. Surgery is usually required in these situations.

In contrast, rectus femoris avulsions require conservative management rather than surgery. This involves minimizing the tension on the muscle by keeping the knee extended as much as possible. Usually, 2 to 3 weeks of rest is necessary before a gradual return to activity is allowed.

Optimally, prompt evaluation of quadriceps strains improves the institution of proper management. RICE is the mainstay of initial management. The compression wrap must be applied from toe to groin to minimize distal edema and the development of deep venous thrombosis. Crutches may be required depending on the extent of disability. After the initial 24 to 72 hours, nonsteroidal anti-inflammatory medications can be administered and physical therapy instituted. This involves pain-free stretching and therapeutic modalities initially, progressing to isometric quadriceps contractions, and advancing to functional rehabilitation as tolerated.

Return to activity can take several days to several weeks depending on the extent and degree of the strain. The athlete must have full range of motion and near full return of strength. Taping or a neoprene sleeve or both may be used for support. Muscle defects may be permanent but do not usually restrict function.

Complications such as retear are not frequent but can occur with inadequate rehabilitation. Myositis ossificans may occur as in a quadriceps contusion. Because the distal femur is a common site for bone tumors in young people, one must investigate the possibility of a tumor if symptoms are out of proportion to the injury or the response to treatment is poor.

Fractures

Similar to hip and pelvic fractures, femur fractures are relatively uncommon in sports. When present they are usually quickly recognized because of the marked pain and deformity. Emergency transfer of the patient to a trauma center is necessary for further evaluation and treatment.

Differential Diagnosis of Hip, Pelvis, or Thigh Pain

Hip and Pelvis Pain

Acute Pain

- ✗ Fracture
- ✗ Muscle strain (adductor, flexor, abductor)
- ✗ Hip pointer
- ✗ Herniated lumbar disk

Chronic Pain

- ✗ Stress fracture
- ✗ Chronic strain (adductor, flexor, abductor)
- ✗ Bursitis (trochanteric, psoas, ischial)
- ✗ Piriformis syndrome
- ✗ Herniated lumbar disk

Thigh Pain

Acute Pain

- ✗ Strain (quadriceps, hamstrings)
- ✗ Contusion
- ✗ Fracture
- ✗ Hip or lumbar pathology

Chronic Pain

- ✗ Chronic strain
- ✗ Myositis ossificans
- ✗ Hip or lumbar pathology

Suggested Readings

Arnheim DD, Prentice WE. Principles of athletic training. 8th ed. St. Louis: CV Mosby, 1993.

Aronen JG, Chronister RD. Quadriceps contusions, hastening the return to play. Phys Sportsmed 1992;20(7):130–136.

Esposito PW. Pelvis, hip and thigh injuries. In: Mellion MB, Walsh WM, Shelton GL, eds. The team physician's handbook. Philadelphia: Hanley and Belfus, 1990:401–413.

Jaivin J, Fox JM. Injuries to the thigh. In: Nicholas JA, Hershman EB, eds. The lower extremity and spine in sports medicine. St. Louis: CV Mosby, 1995:999–1024.

Grana WA, Schelberg-Karnes E. How I manage deep muscle bruises. Phys Sportsmed 1983;11(6):123–127.

Jackson DW, Feagin JA. Quadriceps contusion in young athletes: relation of severity. J Bone Joint Surg 1973;55:95–105.

Lloyd-Smith R, Clement DB, McKenzie DC, et al. A survey of overuse and traumatic hip and pelvic injuries in athletes. Phys Sportsmed 1985;13(10):131–142.

Reid DC. Sports injury assessment and rehabilitation. New York: Churchill Livingstone, 1992.

Renstrom PAFH. Tendon and muscle injuries in the groin area. Clin Sports Med 1992;11:815–831.

Rich BSE, McKeag D. When sciatica is not disk disease, detecting piriformis syndrome in active patients. Phys Sportsmed 1992;20(10):105–115.

Sim FH, Scott SG. Injuries of the pelvis and hip in athletes: anatomy and function. In: Nicholas JA, Hershman EB, eds. The lower extremity and spine in sports medicine. St. Louis: CV Mosby, 1986.

Webber A. Acute soft-tissue injuries in the young athlete. Clin Sports Med 1988;7:611–624.

Weiker GG, Munnings F. How I manage hip and pelvis injuries in adolescents. Phys Sportsmed 1993;21(12):72–82.

Weiker GG, Munnings F. Selected hip and pelvis injuries, managing hip pointers, stress fractures, and more. Phys Sportsmed 1994:22(2):96–106.

CHAPTER 12

Knee Injuries

Eugene E. Berg

Situated between the two longest bones and spanned by the strongest muscles in the body, the knee is subjected to large muscular loads, bending, and rotational moments. Thus this complex joint is vulnerable to injury when stressed in athletic endeavor. The high incidence of knee injuries demands an understanding of its unique anatomy.

Bony Anatomy

The knee is composed of three bones: the femur, tibia, and patella (or knee cap) (Fig. 12.1). The distal femur is composed of two femoral condyles separated by an intercondylar notch. As seen from the side, the femoral condyles are elliptical. The anterior portion of the femoral condyles has a groove that articulates with the patella. The posterior half of the condyles is primarily involved with weight bearing and articulates with the tibia. The intercondylar notch is the site of origin of the two cruciate ligaments. The collateral ligaments are peripheral structures that originate from the femoral epicondyles.

The tibial plateau accepts weight-bearing loads and comprises two communicating compartments. The medial tibial compartment receives approximately 60% of the body's weight in stance, whereas the lateral half accepts 40% of the body's weight. The surface of the tibial plateau is tilted 7° posteriorly, which is equal to the amount the knee is flexed at heel strike, when body weight is transferred to the limb.

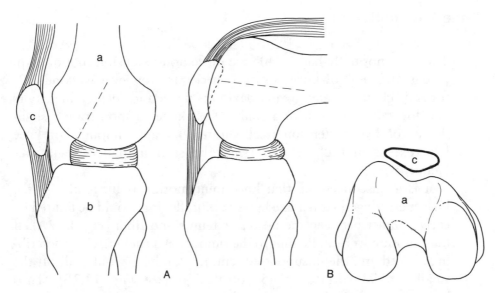

Figure 12.1 *The bony constituents of the knee: the femur (a), tibia (b), and patella (c). (A) The lateral view shows that the femoral condyles are elliptical. (B) In cross section, the patella is triangular and tracks in the anterior (trochlear) groove in the femoral condyles.* (Redrawn by permission from Mueller W. Knee: form, function and ligament reconstruction. New York: Springer Verlag, 1985:82.)

The patella is a triangular bone embedded within the quadriceps muscle (see Fig. 12.1B). It forms a joint with the anterior femoral condyles, elevating the quadriceps muscle from the center of knee rotation and thereby increasing its muscular efficiency. The patella also protects the knee from a direct blow and decreases anterior-posterior tibiofemoral shear stress. Compressive patellofemoral forces are small when the knee is extended and are large during flexion. To dissipate these forces, the area of patellar surface contact with the femur increases with flexion.

The shafts of the femur and tibia are neither parallel nor collinear. The normal alignment of these two bones is angled in 7° of abduction or knock-kneed habitus, also called genu valgum. In general, infants are bowlegged (genu varum) and do not develop the normal knock-kneed valgus alignment until 3 years of age. After that, bowlegs are abnormal and can cause increased medial knee joint loading and accelerated osteoarthritis.

Knee Kinematics

The knee normally has a 140° arc of flexion-extension motion. Approximately 65° of knee flexion is necessary for level walking, 80° for stair climbing, and greater flexion is needed for descending stairs and for getting up out of a chair. Most knees demonstrate a slight degree of hyperextension (recurvatum). Greater amounts of knee hyperextension (10° or more) may be seen in patients with lax ligaments.

It is a misconception that knee joint motion is hinge-like. If the knee were hinged with a fixed pivot point, flexion would be limited by early contact between the posterior femur and tibia (Fig. 12.2A). If knee motion were analogous to the runners of a rocking chair describing a fixed arc, the unsupported femoral condyles would fall off the smaller tibial surface at 45° of flexion (see Fig. 12.2B). Thus knee motion is really a combined synchronous rocking and gliding motion.

As the knee approaches full extension, the femur internally rotates on the tibia. This is called the normal "screw home mechanism," which tightens peripheral ligaments and stabilizes the knee in stance. The medial compartment of the knee, which bears greater weight

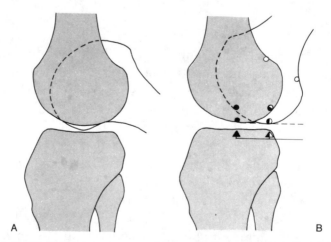

Figure 12.2 *(A) If the knee were a hinge, flexion would be limited to 125° when the tibia and femur would abut. (B) If the knee motion were like the runners on a rocking chair, the femur would rock off of the tibial surface. In actuality, knee motion is a combination of rocking and gliding motions.* (Redrawn by permission from Mueller W. Knee: form, function and ligament reconstruction. Now York: Springer Verlag, 1985:82.)

loads in stance, acts as a pivot point. The lateral half of the knee is more mobile and rotates the femur into a stable posture.

Soft Tissue Anatomy

The bones of the knee joint are geometrically incongruous. Therefore the knee is inherently unstable. Joint stability depends greatly upon the investing soft tissues (principally muscles and ligaments) that cross the joint. As muscles and ligaments are not mineralized like bone, they are not seen on x-rays. They are well seen on magnetic resonance imaging (MRI) scans, however.

The majority of knee joint stability depends on four major knee ligaments (Fig. 12.3): the two peripheral, extra-articular, collateral ligaments, which resist varus and valgus (adduction and abduction) stresses, and the two central intra-articular cruciate ligaments, which restrain abnormal anterior-posterior tibiofemoral stresses. Most musculoskeletal structures do not provide the sole source of joint stability in a given axis of motion. Thus it is important to understand the concept of primary and secondary restraints. Each of the major ligaments provides a primary restraint to abnormal knee motion. However, there are other ligaments (secondary restraints) that confer backup stability and become important when the primary structure has been injured. Specific muscle groups dynamically act as a secondary restraint in a ligament-deficient knee. When appropriately trained and rehabilitated, some muscle groups can compensate for certain injured ligaments.

Intra-articular Ligaments

Cruciate Ligaments

The cruciate ligaments get their name from the Latin word *crucere* because they cross one another (see Fig. 12.3). They are cord-like structures that are named for their tibial attachments. The anterior cruciate ligament (ACL) originates from the inner aspect of the lateral femoral condyle and inserts upon the anterior tibia near the medial meniscus (Fig. 12.4A). The ACL lies within the synovium-lined knee joint cavity. Injury to the ACL is the most frequent cause of a knee hemarthrosis (bloody joint). Joint fluid bathes this ligament and contains enzymes that prevent normal clotting. This may contribute to the fact that the torn ACL heals poorly. The ACL is the primary restraint to anterior translation of the tibia on femur.

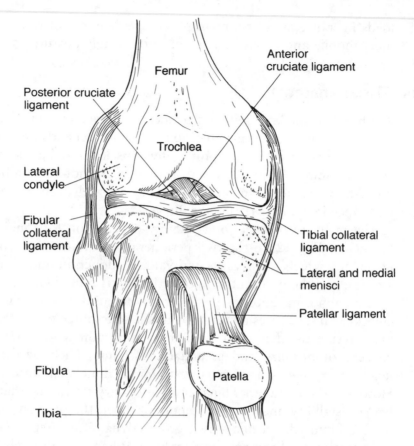

Figure 12.3 *The cruciate (from the Latin* crucere, *for cross) ligaments are intra-articular structures that originate from the intercondylar notch of the femur and insert on the tibia. The peripheral collateral ligaments are extra-articular and surround the joint cavity.* (Redrawn by permission from Hunter-Griffin LY. Athletic training and sports medicine, 2nd ed. Parkridge, IL: AAOS, 1991:317.)

The posterior cruciate ligament (PCL) originates from the medial femoral condyle and inserts upon the posterior tibia behind and below the menisci (see Fig. 12.4B). This ligament is covered by a sheath of synovium. Often when the PCL is ruptured, its synovial sheath will remain intact, and often there will be no hemarthrosis. The PCL is the primary restraint to posterior translation of the tibia on femur.

Menisci

The paired meniscal fibrocartilages are dense structures that are interposed between the femur and tibia. They are C-shaped structures (the

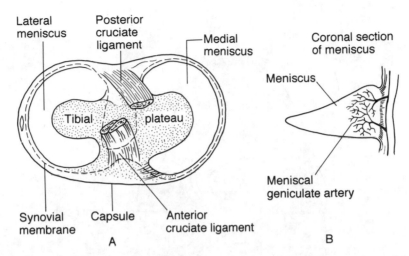

Figure 12.4 *(A) The menisci are interposed between the femoral condyles and tibial plateau. (B) In cross section, the menisci are triangular in shape.* (Redrawn by permission from Hunter-Griffin LY. Athletic training and sports medicine, 2nd ed. Parkridge, IL: AAOS, 1991:317, 362.)

lateral structure is actually almost circular) that deepen the joint and absorb load (see Fig. 12.4). In cross section, the menisci are triangular and act as stabilizing wedges. The peripheral one third of the meniscus is vascular and when torn will mount a healing response. The inner two thirds of the meniscus is avascular and not likely to heal. The menisci absorb and release joint fluid acting as a repository for this source of joint surface nutrition and lubrication. In stance, the anterior portion of the meniscus is loaded when the knee is extended, whereas the posterior meniscus is loaded when the knee is flexed. During flexion, the meniscus is gripped like a cam between the femoral condyles and tibial plateau (see Fig. 12.1). The addition of rotatory stress can cause the meniscus to shear. Whenever there is asynchrony of knee joint flexion and rotation, as when a pivoting athlete arises from a squat, the meniscal fibrocartilage is susceptible to injury. The medial meniscus is more frequently damaged because it is less mobile and bears a greater proportion of body weight than the lateral meniscus. The menisci are vital to proper knee function; even their partial removal hastens the development of arthritic changes.

Synovium

The knee joint is actually a cavity that is lined by a synovial membrane (Fig. 12.5). The synovial membrane is composed of two types

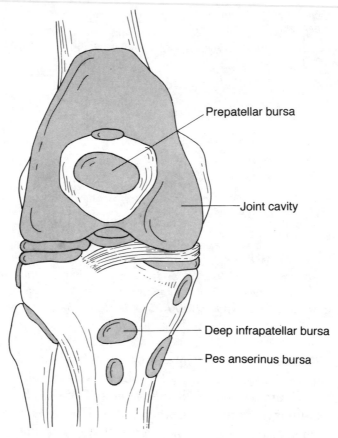

Figure 12.5 *The extent of the synovium-lined cavities around the knee.*
(Redrawn by permission from Fulkerson YP, Hungerford DS. Disorders of the
patellofemoral joint, 2nd ed. Baltimore: Williams and Wilkins, 1990:94.
Copyright © 1990, Williams and Wilkins Co.)

of cells, one removes wear debris, and the other produces large,
complex glycoproteins used to lubricate the moving joint surfaces.
Certain diseases of the immune system, such as rheumatoid arthritis,
cause synovial tissue to thicken, overgrow, and ultimately destroy the
joint. Occasionally synovial hypertrophy occurs after an injury or
joint bleeding.

In some knees, there are synovial septae known as a plica, which
are remnants of incomplete knee joint cavitation during embryonic
development (Fig. 12.6). A potentially troublesome plica, present in
20% of normal knees, originates from the medial patella and extends
to the anterior fat pad of the knee just behind the patellar tendon. A
mediopatellar plica, if enlarged by inflammation, can cause pain when

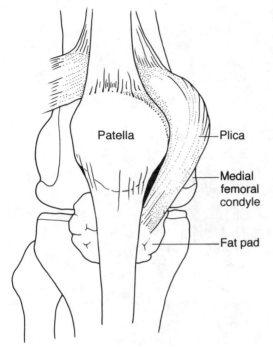

Patella
Plica
Medial femoral condyle
Fat pad

Figure 12.6 *The medial synovial plica is interposed between the patella and the medial femoral condyle.* (Redrawn by permission from Hunter-Griffin LY. Athletic training and sports medicine, 2nd ed. Parkridge, IL: AAOS, 1991:320.)

it is trapped between the patella and the medial femoral condyle during knee flexion.

Extra-articular Ligaments

Collateral Ligaments

The medial collateral ligament resists valgus (abduction) knee stress. Divided into superficial and deep components, the superficial medial collateral ligament is the major restraint to valgus loads. It is a stout, expansive structure that originates from the medial femoral epicondyle, is widest at the joint line, and has a broad insertion on the proximal tibia (Fig. 12.7). The superficial medial collateral ligament slides posteriorly with flexion. Its anterior fibers remain tight in all knee positions, whereas the posterior fibers relax with flexion. The deep medial collateral ligament, sometimes called the coronary ligament, is divided into anterior, middle, and posterior thirds and secures the meniscus to bone. It is also known as the meniscofemoral and meniscotibial ligaments. The posterior third of the deep MCL is also described as the posterior oblique ligament.

The lateral collateral ligament is cord-like and smaller than the medial collateral ligament. It extends from the lateral femoral

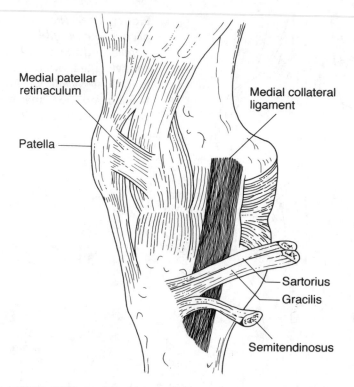

Figure 12.7 *The medial side of the knee.* (Redrawn by permission from Hunter-Griffin LY. Athletic training and sports medicine, 2nd ed. Parkridge, IL: AAOS, 1991:321.)

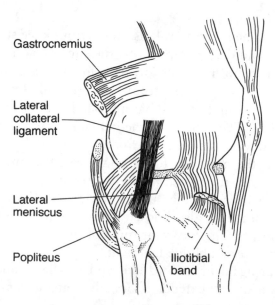

Figure 12.8 *The lateral knee ligament complex.* (Redrawn by permission from Hunter-Griffin LY. Athletic training and sports medicine, 2nd ed. Parkridge, IL: AAOS, 1991:323.)

epicondyle and inserts upon the fibular head (Fig. 12.8). This ligament confers 70% of the knee's opposition to varus (adduction) stress. The arcuate ligament is a deep capsular ligament located posterior to the lateral collateral that together with the popliteus muscle helps to control external rotation of the tibia.

Patellar Retinaculum

The medial patellar retinaculum is a collagenous structure that attaches the medial border of the patella to the medial femoral condyle and knee joint capsule (see Fig. 12.7). Its function is to centralize the patella and hold it medially. The retinaculum resists the tendency of the patella to slip laterally because of the valgus relation of the femur and tibia.

Muscle

Medial Muscles

The tendons of three muscles (sartorius, gracilis, and semitendinosus) cross the superficial medial collateral ligament to insert upon the medial tibia (Fig. 12.9). These muscles provide a small secondary restraint to valgus stress and external rotation. The semimembranosus, semitendinosus, gracilis, and biceps femoris are known as the hamstring muscles and act to flex the knee. Secondarily they aid the anterior cruciate ligament in preventing anterior tibial translation.

Lateral Muscles

The iliotibial tract originates from the tensor fascia lata and gluteus maximus muscle and extends over the lateral thigh (Fig. 12.10). At knee level an anterior segment inserts upon the patella, which it stabilizes. The posterior iliotibial tract fibers insert upon an anterolateral tibial prominence called Gerdy's tubercle (see Fig. 12.10). The biceps femoris is the lateral hamstring muscle, which also flexes the knee. Its tendon inserts upon the fibular head. The iliotibial tract and to a lesser extent the biceps femoris are secondary lateral stabilizers.

Just posterior and distal to the biceps femoris tendon is the peroneal nerve, which wraps around the fibular neck. The peroneal nerve is vulnerable to traction injuries from severe adduction knee trauma. A peroneal nerve palsy combined with a lateral knee injury is worri-

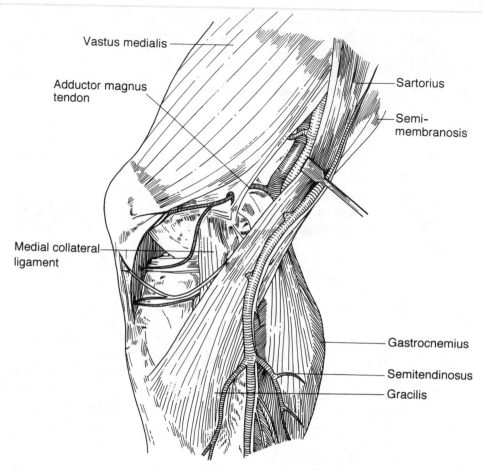

Figure 12.9 *Medial muscles of the knee.* (Redrawn by permission from Insall JN. Surgery of the knee. New York: Churchill Livingstone, 1984:5.)

some. This combination is associated with devastating soft tissue injuries that involve not only the lateral collateral ligament but also one or more of the cruciate ligaments.

Anterior Muscles

The quadriceps, as the name suggests, comprises four components: vastus medius, vastus lateralis, vastus intermedius, and rectus femoris (Fig. 12.11). It is an antigravity muscle, responsible for knee extension. Two of the four muscles, the vastus intermedius and rectus femoris, become tendinous as they insert on the superior patellar pole and compose the quadriceps tendon. The vastus medialis muscle inserts upon the medial patella, contributes little to knee extension, but is a patellar stabilizer that counteracts the tendency for the patella

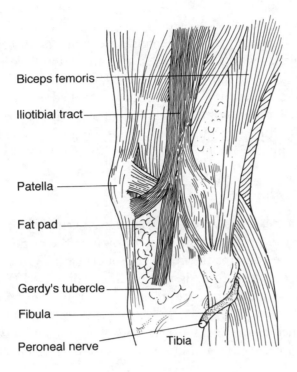

Figure 12.10 *The lateral knee musculature.* (Redrawn by permission from Hunter-Griffin LY. Athletic training and sports medicine, 2nd ed. Parkridge, IL: AAOS, 1991:323.)

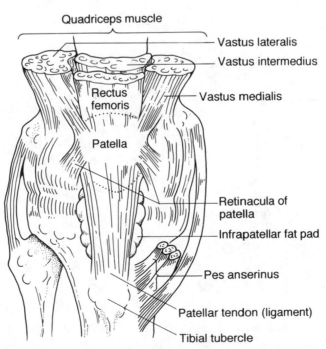

Figure 12.11 *Anterior knee musculature.* (Redrawn by permission from Hunter-Griffin LY. Athletic training and sports medicine, 2nd ed. Parkridge, IL: AAOS, 1991:321.)

to subluxate laterally in early flexion owing to the valgus femorotibial axis. The patella is enveloped by fascial expanses from the quadriceps muscle, called retinacula, which extend medially and laterally onto the femoral epicondyles and centralize the patella in the trochlear groove of the femur. Inferiorly the patella is embedded in a thick tendon (the patellar tendon) that inserts upon the tibial tuberosity. As an anterior structure, the quadriceps acts synergistically with the posterior cruciate ligament to prevent posterior tibial translation.

Posterior Muscles

The horizontal flexion crease at the back of the knee is actually almost 5 cm proximal to the tibiofemoral joint line. Known as the popliteal fossa, the posterior knee contains the important neurovascular structures of the leg. The popliteal fossa is shaped like a diamond (Fig. 12.12). The superior boundaries are formed by the hamstring muscles: the biceps femoris muscle laterally; the semimembranosus and semitendinosus medially. The inferior boundary is defined by the two heads of the gastrocnemius muscle, which originate from the

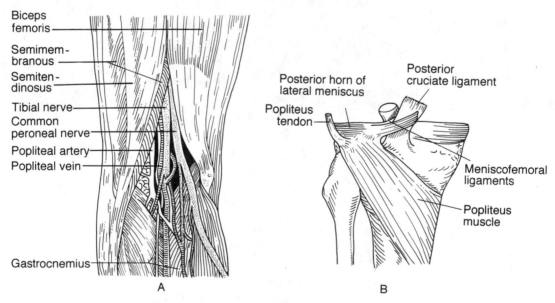

Figure 12.12 *The posterior knee: superficial layer (A) and deep layer (B).* (Part A redrawn by permission from Hunter-Griffin LY. Athletic training and sports medicine, 2nd ed. Parkridge, IL: AAOS, 1991:321. Part B redrawn by permission from Campbell. Operative orthopedics, 8th ed. St. Louis: Mosby, 1991:1505.)

posterior femoral condyles. Deep to the gastrocnemius is the popliteus muscle, an internal rotator of the tibia that inserts upon three lateral structures: the fibular head, the lateral meniscus, and the femoral condyle just anterior to the lateral collateral ligament. The popliteus tendon, the arcuate (posterior lateral capsular) ligament, and the lateral head of the gastrocnemius have been called the arcuate complex (see Fig. 12.8). The semimembranosus muscle reinforces the posterior knee joint capsule with an expansion called the popliteal oblique ligament and also attaches to the medial meniscus and tibia (see Fig. 12.9). The popliteal artery and the tibial nerve reside deep in the popliteal fossa lying superficial to the popliteus muscle. The peroneal nerve diverges from the tibial nerve and runs with the biceps femoris tendon (see Fig. 12.12). It is subcutaneous beneath the fibular head, where it is vulnerable to direct injury.

Injury Evaluation and Treatment

Ligaments are collagenous structures that attach one bone to another, restrain the joint from abnormal motion, and thus act to guide normal motion. A sprain is a ligament injury and is classified as one of three types depending upon its severity. A grade I sprain implies that there has been microscopic ligament damage yet the ligament maintains full structural integrity. On examination, a ligament that has sustained a grade I injury will be tender to palpation and manual stress but will be stable to applied stress. A grade II sprain implies a more severe injury in which the ligament fibers have experienced some structural elongation. The ligament will be in gross continuity but will exhibit increased laxity when stress tested. The most severe, grade III injury causes a total disruption of ligament structure. The ligament is discontinuous and will demonstrate overt instability when stressed. This grading system is discussed in more detail in Chapter 2. In general, the contralateral, uninjured limb is readily available as a control for stress test comparison. This is particularly helpful when examining the flexible athlete with constitutionally lax ligaments.

On the field or at courtside, a brief history should be obtained to describe the mechanism of injury. As there will be an early period of transient anesthesia after injury, a quick attempt should be made to ascertain the degree of knee instability. It is important to check distal arterial pulses to exclude a limb-threatening injury to the blood supply. The joint should then be splinted, wounds should be sterilely dressed, and the patient should be prepared for transport to a treating facility.

Acute Injuries

Anterior Cruciate Ligament Injuries

The anterior cruciate ligament (ACL) is the most commonly injured knee ligament in athletes. An intra-articular structure, it is also the most frequent cause of acute knee hemarthrosis. Approximately 70% of the patients who have a bloody knee effusion will have demonstrable damage to the ACL.

Mechanism

Five mechanisms are known to cause an ACL injury.

1. The roof of the intercondylar notch of the femur can amputate the ACL in hyperextension.
2. A direct blow to the posterior aspect of the leg that drives the tibia anterior may shear the ACL.
3. The ACL provides backup restraint for varus and valgus stress. It can be injured secondarily but only after the collateral ligament has failed (Fig. 12.13).
4. The ACL may fail with violent internal rotation of the tibia on the femur, especially in athletes with narrow intercondylar notches. This mechanism may occur in a noncontact mode (e.g., pivoting) and is associated with a painful popping, a hemarthrosis, and subsequent giving way.
5. Finally, the ACL can fail in hyperflexion with an intense co-contraction of the quadriceps muscle. This type of injury is seen in elite skiers whose center of gravity falls behind their skis with a loss of balance. To prevent the impending fall, they violently contract their quadriceps muscle, which forces the tibia anteriorly. The ACL then fails under tension caused by knee flexion and quadriceps-induced shear.

Diagnosis

Injury to the intra-articular ACL will cause it to bleed into the joint. A bloody knee effusion that occurred soon after injury is presumptive evidence that the ACL has been injured.

Three tests are used to diagnose an ACL injury. The anterior drawer test and Lachman's test detect increased amounts of anterior

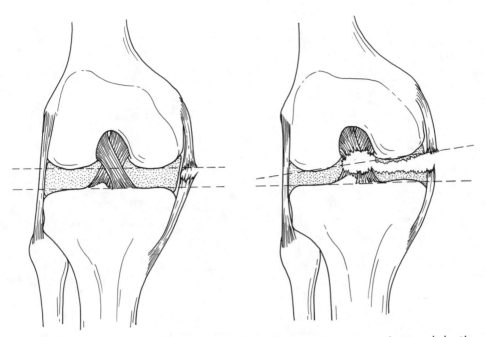

Figure 12.13 *The medial collateral ligament is the primary restraint to abduction or valgus stress. When injurious forces are large, the cruciate ligaments may also be torn in their role as secondary restraints to valgus loading.* (Redrawn by permission from Mueller W. Knee: form, function and ligament reconstruction. New York: Springer Verlag, 1985;141.)

tibial translation on the femur. The anterior drawer test is generally well known but unfortunately not a very sensitive test. In the drawer maneuver, the athlete is supine and the knee is flexed 90°. The examiner secures the foot by sitting on it. The examiner's thumbs are placed on the joint line, and the tibia is pulled anteriorly (Fig. 12.14). The hamstring muscle must be relaxed. Abnormal motion is compared with motion on the normal side and is graded on a four plus (++++) scale. Each plus sign represents 0.5 cm of increased laxity. For example, a three plus (+++) anterior drawer would signify 1.5 cm of greater anterior tibial displacement than that of the uninjured side.

Often the drawer test is negative because of a bloody joint effusion, pain, and capsular tightness. Lachman's test is a similar maneuver done with the knee in 30° of flexion. The proximal tibia is grasped with one hand and the distal femur is stabilized with the other as anterior translatory stress is applied to the tibia. In 30° of flexion meniscal geometry is less constraining and the collateral ligaments are

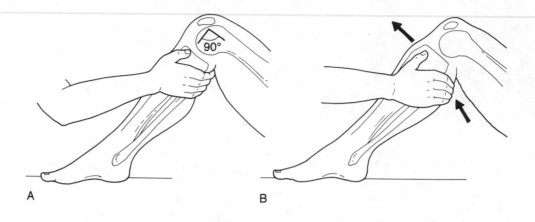

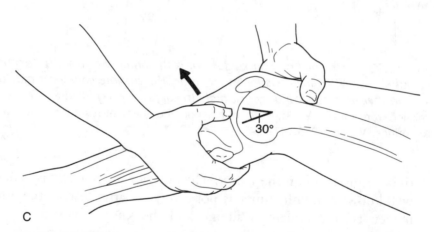

Figure 12.14 *(A) The anterior drawer test. (B) Lachman's maneuver.* (Redrawn by permission from Hunter-Griffin LY. Athletic training and sports medicine, 2nd ed. Parkridge, IL: AAOS, 1991:337.)

relaxed. Lachman's 30° position facilitates the detection of very subtle side-to-side joint laxity differences and is generally preferred over the anterior drawer test.

The pivot shift test is difficult to perform acutely in an apprehensive patient who guards a painful, swollen knee. It cannot be elicited when there is a knee flexion contracture from either a displaced meniscus tear or a large joint effusion. Despite these problems, when the test is positive, it is very specific for ACL dysfunction. The pivot shift test detects tibiofemoral subluxation. It can be elicited using a variety of techniques with confusing eponyms (e.g., the Slocum, Losee, Hughston, jerk, and MacIntosh tests). All demonstrate the tibiofemoral subluxation that occurs because of an incompetent ACL. An easy method of performing the pivot shift test is to place the knee in full extension and maximal internal tibial rotation. The examiner holds the lateral leg close to his or her body and applies valgus stress by leaning into the joint. A positive test will produce a sudden jump of the knee as it is flexed. In the position of extension with internal tibial rotation, the tibia is subluxated on the femur. As flexion is initiated, one feels the clunk of the reduction. Often the patient will confirm that this maneuver reproduces the giving way sensation that he or she experiences (Fig. 12.15).

The ACL is rarely injured in isolation. In almost 50% of cases there will be concomitant damage to one or both of the menisci. MRI scans have shown there to be a high incidence of subclinical injuries to bone and articular cartilage that are not detectable by radiographs. The concomitant injury to the joint surface and its underlying bony support contributes to the accelerated arthritis known to occur after an ACL injury.

Natural History

Untreated athletes can respond in one of three ways to their ACL-deficient knee. Some will voluntarily restrict their activities and switch to less demanding sports. These individuals will function well with a

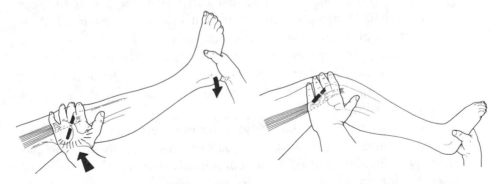

Figure 12.15 *The pivot shift test for anterior cruciate ligament deficiency. The knee is fully extended and maximally internally rotated. Then a valgus stress is applied by leaning into the knee. In this position, the tibia is subluxated on the femur. At 20° to 30° of flexion, the knee will reduce with a jump.* (Redrawn by permission from Losee RE. The pivot shift. In: Feagin JA, ed. The crucial ligaments. New York: Churchill Livingstone, 1988:309.)

neuromuscular rehabilitation program and functional bracing. Others will reduce their activity levels and tolerate infrequent episodes of instability. Finally, a large number of patients experience repeated knee giving way that significantly affects the quality of their lives and is debilitating. The latter are candidates for ligament reconstruction.

Thus nonoperative treatment can be beneficial for the low-demand, recreational athlete whose sport does not require much twisting, jumping, and change of direction. Gymnastics, volleyball, and basketball are sports that place the ACL at great risk of injury. An ACL injury is often career-ending in these sports, as recurrent knee instability is incompatible with competitive performance.

Treatment

After a brief examination (on the field) to establish a tentative diagnosis and check the neurovascular status of the limb, the knee should be iced and splinted. The athlete should be placed on crutches and allowed to bear weight on the limb only for balance. A hemarthrosis indicates that a significant joint injury has occurred and should prompt a referral to someone capable of rendering definitive treatment.

Initial nonoperative treatment involves temporary immobilization of the knee in a brace for both comfort and protection. Early joint motion is allowed after the initial swelling and pain have subsided to prevent joint contracture, but the emphasis of early treatment is to protect the injured joint from further disruptive stresses. If the secondary stabilizers are also injured, weight bearing is restricted. At 6 weeks, the healing process is sufficiently advanced in the secondary stabilizers to permit weight bearing. If the secondary stabilizers (collateral ligaments, menisci) appear intact, both weight-bearing and motion exercises are advanced more quickly, guided by the patient's pain and swelling.

The hamstring knee flexor muscles act in synergy with the ACL to prevent anterior tibial translation. Gait studies have shown that patients with incompetent ACLs subconsciously increase the amount of knee flexion in all activities. Flexion enhances the action of the hamstring muscles in controlling anterior tibial shear. Thus most nonoperative ACL treatment protocols emphasize compensatory hamstring muscle strengthening. Normally hamstring muscle strength is only 70% that of the stronger antigravity quadriceps muscle. The goal of muscular rehabilitation is to have the hamstring muscles on the ACL-injured side equal the measured strength of the strongest quadriceps.

Functional knee bracing has a controversial role in nonoperative treatment. While many braces do not significantly restrict the amount of anterior tibial translation in the ACL-deficient knee, the 10° extension stop can prevent tibiofemoral pivot shift subluxation. The brace may also provide the athlete with proprioceptive information. There has been some success with neuromuscular biofeadback and proprioception training programs in which ACL-deficient athletes are taught compensatory techniques to prevent the knee from giving way. In general, nonoperative treatment is most successful in low-demand individuals with tight secondary restraining ligaments. It is probably the treatment of choice in children, in whom surgery can cause growth disturbances of the femur and tibia.

Operative treatment is indicated for individuals who have failed rehabilitation and experience frequent knee joint instability. Certain occupations rely upon a good sense of balance and may require ligament reconstruction to ensure employee safety.

When the ligament is avulsed from either its bony origin or insertion, surgical reattachment is successful. However, most ACL tears occur within the substance of the ligament. The results of direct sutured repair of interstitial cruciate ligament tears have been unpredictable and disappointing. Thus midsubstance ACL tears are usually reconstructed with tissue substitutes such as the hamstring or patellar tendon. The tissue can be obtained from the patient (autograft) or can be transplanted from a cadaveric donor (allograft).

Anterior cruciate ligament reconstruction has proved to be a very effective surgical procedure that can dependably eliminate the pivot shift and repeated episodes of giving way in 85% to 90% of all cases. It is doubtful, however, that even the best reconstruction will ever attain the properties of the uninjured native ligament.

Posterior Cruciate Ligament

Mechanism

Unlike the anterior cruciate ligament, which may be injured in a noncontact mode, the posterior cruciate ligament is usually damaged in violent, high kinetic energy injuries. The mechanism usually involves a blow to the anterior leg such as with a dashboard injury. Posterior cruciate ligament injuries often occur in combination with fractures, specifically to the patella and hip, or in combination with other knee ligament injuries. It is unusual for the PCL to be injured in isolation. The PCL can also fail as a secondary stabilizer to varus and valgus stress after the collateral ligament has been ruptured (see Fig. 12.13). Popliteal artery damage often occurs with PCL injuries. Thus it is essential to evaluate the status of this artery. In young patients with a normal circulatory system, any palpable asymmetry in pulses is an emergency and demands an arteriogram. It is unconscionable to theorize that the diminution of lower extremity pulses is due to arterial "spasm."

Diagnosis

The tests used to evaluate the PCL assess posterior tibial translation on the femur. The posterior drawer test is done with the patient supine, the knee flexed 90°, and the foot stabilized similar to the starting position of the anterior drawer test. The examiner's hands are placed on the joint line as the tibia is pushed posteriorly on the femur. Increased posterior translation compared with that on the uninjured side indicates a PCL injury and is graded in 0.5-cm increments. The gravity drop back test is done with the patient supine, with hips and knees flexed 90°. With an absent or elongated PCL, gravity will pull the tibia posteriorly. This is detected visually by noting tibial sag or the decreased prominence of the tibial tuberosity anteriorly (Fig. 12.16).

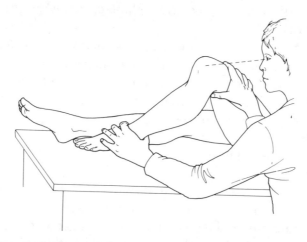

Figure 12.16 *The gravity drop back test. With the knee flexed 70° to 90°, the absence of a posterior cruciate ligament will allow the tibia to subluxate posteriorly.* (Redrawn by permission from Poss R. Orthopaedic knowledge update, 3nd ed. Parkridge, IL: AAOS, 1990:558.)

Natural History

Isolated PCL incompetence is reasonably well tolerated. Unless the patient has a bowed (varus) knee, the complaint of instability and giving way is unusual. More frequently patients complain of anterior patellofemoral pain associated with activities that require active knee flexion such as stair climbing, squatting, or arising from a chair. The quadriceps muscle and the PCL are agonist structures, both acting to maintain an anterior tibial position relative to the femur. In the absence of a PCL, the quadriceps muscle must compensate to maintain proper tibiofemoral alignment. This places an increased load upon the patellofemoral joint, which causes pain and may accelerate arthritic changes.

Treatment

The acute management of the PCL is similar to that of any injured ligament. The painful knee is placed at rest by splinting and decreased weight bearing. Ice is used to minimize swelling and to afford analgesia.

Athletes with very strong quadriceps muscles have been capable of high-level competitive athletic performance without an intact PCL. Thus rehabilitation should focus upon compensatory strengthening of the quadriceps. There are currently no reliable bracing systems that prevent posterior translation of the tibia on the femur.

As the incidence of PCL injury is small, so too is the experience with operative treatment. If the ligament is disrupted at its bony origin or insertion, acute surgical repair is often successful. Similar to the anterior cruciate ligament, the results of intrasubstance PCL repair have been disappointing. This type of injury is best reconstructed with substitute tissue. Arthroscopic methods of PCL reconstruction with stout allogenic and autogenic collagenous material have been perfected and have given promising results.

Medial Collateral Ligament

Mechanism

As the primary medial knee stabilizer, the medial collateral ligament is typically injured from an abduction or valgus stress to the knee. Severe grade III injuries to this ligament are often associated with concomitant cruciate ligament and meniscal pathology (see Fig. 12.13).

Diagnosis

A damaged ligament will be tender to direct palpation at the site of rupture, which can be anywhere between its origin from the prominence of the medial femoral epicondyle to its insertion upon the medial tibia. Diffuse, acute knee swelling without a contained knee effusion is an ominous sign. It suggests that the deep capsular, meniscofemoral, or meniscotibial ligaments have been disrupted, which has allowed blood and joint fluid to leak into the soft tissues.

The application of valgus knee stress will reproduce discomfort and may demonstrate increased laxity (Fig. 12.17). Abduction (valgus) stress testing should be done with the knee in full extension, as well as in 30° of flexion. In slight flexion, the posterior joint capsule and cruciate ligaments are somewhat relaxed. Geometrically, the knee is less stable in slight flexion, as the femoral condyles, menisci, and tibial joint surfaces are not congruously aligned. Thus more subtle degrees of laxity of the collateral ligaments will be

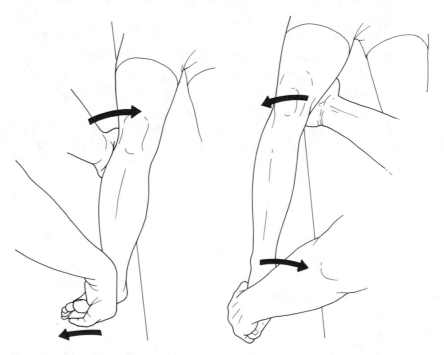

Figure 12.17 *Abduction (valgus) and abduction (varus) stress tests are used to assess the integrity of the medial and lateral collateral ligaments, respectively.* (Redrawn by permission from Hunter-Griffin LY. Athletic training and sports medicine, 2nd ed. Parkridge, IL: AAOS, 1991:337.)

exhibited when stress testing is done under a slight amount of knee flexion. Abduction laxity with the knee in the more stable, fully extended posture implies a greater magnitude of injury, which may include injury to the posterior knee joint capsule and cruciate ligaments. Abduction or valgus stress testing is usually done with the examiner's digits placed on the joint line and is estimated in millimeters of increased joint space opening or degrees of laxity when compared with the normal side. If the joint space opening is greater than 1 cm, it is likely that one of the cruciate ligaments is also involved.

Treatment

When injured in isolation, if the torn ligament ends are not widely separated, the medial collateral ligament will heal well when protected from stress. This injury can be definitively treated in a long leg cast or a rehabilitation brace, hinged at the knee. It is important to determine whether or not there has been a simultaneous injury to a cruciate ligament because the medial collateral ligament may not heal as tightly as needed when the secondary restraining force of the cruciate ligament is absent. A torn cruciate ligament cannot "protect" the healing collateral ligament, and a healed but lax ligament results. In questionable cases, arthroscopy or MRI may be required to evaluate the status of the cruciate ligaments and menisci.

Mild forms of medial collateral injury without significant laxity (grade I sprains) may be managed symptomatically. Isometric muscle strengthening and mobilization are started as soon as the symptoms allow. Once the athlete is able to ambulate without a limp, running straight ahead on level ground is allowable. When the athlete can run without a limp, cutting is permitted. When quadriceps and hamstring muscle strength approach the strength of the normal side, competitive activities and light contact are permissible. Many team physicians believe that prophylactic knee braces are most effective in protecting the athlete who has sustained and is recovering from an isolated medial collateral ligament injury.

Operative treatment is best reserved for patients in whom the medial collateral ligament is injured in combination with other knee ligaments.

Lateral Collateral Ligament

Injury to the lateral collateral ligament results from a varus or adduction stress to the knee. This can occur when an athlete is struck on the medial aspect of the knee. Patients with bowlegs may be predisposed to this type of injury. The lateral collateral ligament may also be injured by severe external rotation of the tibia.

Diagnosis

The athlete is tender over the lateral collateral ligament, anywhere between the lateral femoral epicondyle and the fibular head. With the examiner's fingers placed on the joint line, the amount of lateral joint space widening is palpated when varus stress is applied. The knee should be tested for varus instability with the knee in both 0° and 30° of knee joint flexion (see Fig. 12.17). Laxity with the knee in full extension implies a greater degree of soft tissue damage (such as concomitant cruciate injury) than if laxity can be detected only in the 30° flexed position. Comparison with the normal side is helpful in determining the relative magnitude of the injury to the ligament. Injury to the arcuate ligament complex, iliotibial tract, the popliteus and biceps femoris tendons, as well as the peroneal nerve, can occur with lateral-side injuries. A peroneal nerve palsy, almost always associated with tears of one or both cruciate ligaments, is manifest by dorsal foot numbness and toe and ankle extensor weakness.

The lateral collateral ligament and arcuate complex resist external rotation of the tibia on the femur. These structures are examined by evaluation of passive external tibial rotation (Fig. 12.18). External rotatory instability of the knee can be determined by measuring the maximum passive external tibial rotation of the tibia and foot. External tibial rotation should be described with the knee at 90° as well as at 30° of flexion. The latter position is reported to be more sensitive to changes in tibial rotation. Asymmetry of external tibial rotation of more than 20° suggests an injury to the lateral collateral ligament, arcuate ligament, and popliteal tendon complex.

Treatment

Acutely the knee is managed with ice, immobilization, protected motion, and weight bearing. Similar to the medial collateral ligament, nonoperative treatment is indicated when the lateral collateral ligament–arcuate complex is injured in isolation. With a concomitant cruciate ligament injury, the lateral ligament structures may be repaired at the time of cruciate ligament surgery. In bowlegged athletes with varus knees, a tibial osteotomy is sometimes necessary

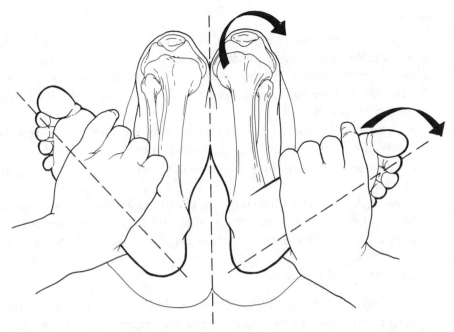

Figure 12.18 *Testing of the posterolateral ligament complex. Incompetence of the lateral collateral ligament and arcuate complex allows for increased external tibial rotation.* (Redrawn by permission from Loomer RL. A test for knee postereolateral rotary instability. Clin Orth Op 1991;264:236–237.)

to decrease normal adduction stresses to the injured lateral soft tissues.

Peroneal nerve dysfunction is a clue to the severity of injury and should cause one to be suspicious of a cruciate ligament injury and knee dislocation. Pulses must be checked, and if they are diminished, referral should be made emergently.

Knee Dislocation

A knee dislocation results from an injury to two or more ligaments at the same time. Only with this degree of ligament disruption can the joint surfaces of the femur and tibia be completely dissociated. The dislocation is named after the direction of tibial displacement (e.g., a posterior knee dislocation describes the tibia to be posteriorly disengaged from the femur). Knee dislocations are usually caused by high-velocity trauma that can also injure the bone and neurovascular structures.

Treatment

Evaluation of limb vascularity is critical! Every documented knee dislocation demands an anatomic study of the popliteal artery on an arteriogram. Injury to the popliteal artery demands an emergent vascular reconstruction to save the limb, before any ligamentous treatment is initiated.

A knee dislocation is reduced with manual traction and pressure to return the limb to its normal alignment. Rarely, interposed tissue can prevent joint relocation. In this instance surgery is required to reduce the knee.

Knee dislocations ultimately require extensive ligament reconstruction and repair. Even under the most favorable circumstances, some knee motion is lost and premature arthritis can develop.

Meniscal Injury

In stance, more than 60% of the body's weight is carried on the peripheral aspect of the tibial plateau by the meniscal fibrocartilages. The remaining 40% is borne by the central portion of the tibial joint surface. In younger persons, meniscal injuries are often concurrent with ligament injuries. The normal aging process causes the menisci to lose resiliency. Thus in older athletes the menisci are more likely to be injured in isolation. The menisci are pinched, cam-like, by the femoral condyle and tibial plateau as the knee flexes. When a rotatory, twisting stress is added, the trapped menisci can tear centrifugally. Meniscal tears in older persons usually occur horizontally within the substance of the meniscus (Fig. 12.19). Younger persons more often tear a meniscus at its synovial junction near the capsular border. As the peripheral portion of the meniscus is vascular, these tears are likely to heal if repaired.

When a meniscal tear is extensive, the torn segment can displace into the joint and cause a mechanical block that prevents full knee motion. A block to terminal knee extension or flexion is called "locking." Patients often describe a self-learned method of unlocking the knee in which the joint is placed in a non-weight-bearing position and is then flexed, extended, and rotated passively. This maneuver may dislodge the displaced meniscus and allow the sudden resumption of full motion. A flap tear of the posterior meniscus can cause giving way as the meniscus loses its stabilizing, doorstop effect with the knee in flexion. A torn meniscus can cause chronic knee swelling and pain as

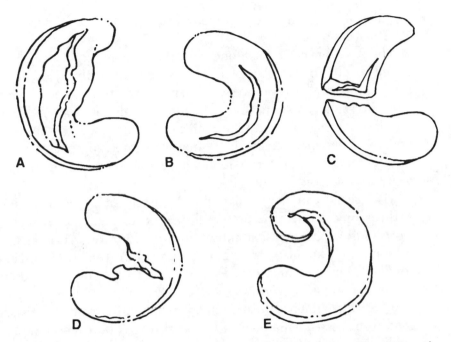

Figure 12.19 *Arthroscopic terminology for meniscal tear configuration: the bucket handle tear is a large longitudinal peripheral tear (AB); the degenerative or horizontal tear (C); a vertical or radial tear (D); a flap tear (E). (Reproduced by permission from Richmond J, Shahady E. Sports medicine for primary care. Cambridge, MA: Blackwell Science, 1995.)*

it injuries the joint surface or can directly irritate the synovium. Meniscal injuries, especially of long duration, can result in an arthritic joint surface.

Diagnosis

Interposed between the femur and tibia, the menisci are palpable in the indented joint space between these two bones. Joint line tenderness is found in more than 50% of bonafide meniscal injuries. Joint line tenderness is specific for a meniscal injury even when a collateral ligament has been injured.

McMurray's tests is used to detect a tear of the meniscus that can be displaced. The test is performed by flexing and extending the knee between 90° and 140° of flexion. One of the examiner's hands rotates the tibia at the ankle while the other hand is placed on the joint line. This is followed by extension of the knee in the rotated position.

A palpable click indicates an unstable tear of the meniscus (Fig. 12.20).

The Apley grind test is done with the patient prone and the knee flexed to 60° to 90°. An axial load is applied to the tibia, directed toward the femur to compress the menisci. The tibia is then internally and externally rotated. Reproduction of pain or a palpable click signifies a meniscal tear. The tear can be localized to the anterior portion of the meniscus if the symptoms or clicking occurs with the knee extended. A posterior meniscal tear will be evident in greater degrees of flexion.

MRI scans can help make the diagnosis of a meniscal lesion. Arthroscopy is often the preferred method of diagnosis if there is a strong suspicion because it allows not only for direct visualization of the pathology but also for definitive surgical treatment. Meniscal tear configuration has implications for both treatment and outcome. Spoke-like radial or vertical tears are perpendicular to the meniscus (see Fig. 12.19). These tears extend peripherally from the avascular central meniscus. This type of meniscal tear is best resected, as it is unlikely to heal. Longitudinal tears parallel the circumference of the meniscus. When this type of tear is peripheral in the vascularized zone, it is amenable to repair. Bucket handle tears are large longitudinal tears and, like the handle of a bucket, can be flipped to either side of the joint. The bucket handle meniscus tear causes locking (prevention of full knee flexion or extension) when displaced. Degenerative or horizontal tears occur within the substance of the meniscus and may not be seen directly from the meniscal surface. These tears usually are associated with underlying arthritis and require resection.

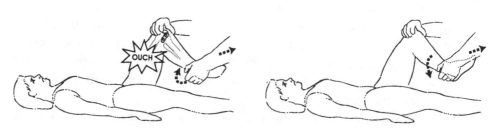

Figure 12.20 *McMurray's test. The examiner places his or her fingers over the joint line of the flexed knee while applying a rotatory force upon the tibia. The knee is subsequently extended in this position. A painful pop constitutes a positive test.* (Reproduced by permission from Richmond J, Shahady E. Sports medicine for primary care. Cambridge, MA: Blackwell Science, 1995.)

Treatment

An isolated meniscal injury without ligament instability can be managed nonoperatively when it is torn peripherally in its vascular zone and is stable. Meniscal healing is likely to occur if the knee is protected from rotatory stresses.

Arthroscopic surgery is indicated if the knee is irreducibly locked in either flexion or extension. Arthroscopic evaluation is also warranted with recurrent knee swelling, locking, giving way, or when joint line pain is refractory to nonoperative treatment. Unstable meniscal tears in the outer third near the synovial junction have excellent healing potential and should be repaired. Meniscal repair does require postoperative protection and temporary immobilization. The success of meniscal repair is compromised when the anterior cruciate ligament has been damaged, as abnormal joint kinematics and recurrent tibiofemoral subluxation subject the repair to increased stress, resulting in failure to heal.

Meniscal tears in the avascular, inner two thirds, as well as degenerative horizontal cleavage tears, are unlikely to heal. In these situations a partial meniscectomy is preferred, in which just the irreparably torn meniscal segment is resected, leaving a stable rim of meniscal tissue. All effort is made to preserve as much stable meniscus as possible, to minimize the likelihood of postmeniscectomy arthritis. Rehabilitation from a partial meniscectomy can be rapid, and immediate motion and exercises are permissible following the surgery.

Discoid Meniscus

The normal meniscus is horseshoe-shaped, with a central absence of fibrocartilage. The discoid meniscus results from a failure of the central meniscal tissue to resorb during embryonic development. Thus the discoid meniscus is a solid disk of fibrocartilage. There is an increased incidence of discoid menisci in Orientals, most often affecting the lateral meniscus. Most discoid menisci are at no greater risk of injury than their normal counterparts. Tears of discoid menisci are amenable to partial arthroscopic meniscectomy. Discoid menisci that have deficient capsular, muscular, and ligamentous attachments are hypermobile and may cause asymptomatic clicking in children. The surgical treatment of the symptomatic hypermobile discoid meniscal tears can be problematic.

Patellar Instability

Embedded in the quadriceps muscle, the patella acts to increase the efficiency of that muscle as it extends the knee. Because the normal knee is in slightly knock-kneed or valgus alignment, the patellar tendon angles laterally relative to the direction of pull of the quadriceps muscle (Fig. 12.21). This is described as the Q (quadriceps) angle, which is normally less than 15°, and results in a laterally directed force on the patella with the initial flexion. Femoral internal rotation, or anteversion, and tibial external rotation accentuate the Q angle and predispose one to patellar malalignment and lateral instability.

The patella may be totally displaced (dislocated) or partially displaced (subluxated) from the femoral groove by either a direct blow or an excessive muscular contraction. Simultaneous knee flexion and external rotation may cause the patella to dislocate laterally. The patient will describe the dislocation as "giving way." Subluxation implies a transient phenomenon in which the patella will spontaneously reduce. Sometimes the athlete or coach will grab the lateral knee and apply medial pressure to the patella, which with simultaneous knee extension will cause the dislocation to reduce. Patellar instability is common in women because their broader pelvis increases their

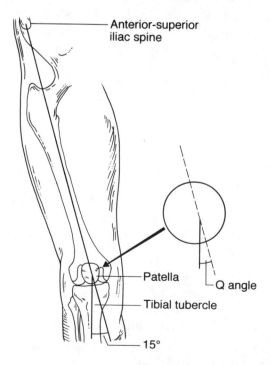

Anterior-superior iliac spine

Patella

Tibial tubercle

Q angle

15°

Figure 12.21 *The tibia and femur are normally in slight valgus alignment resulting in a Q angle between the quadriceps pull and patellar tendon.* (Redrawn by permission from Hunter-Griffin LY. Athletic training in sports medicine, 2nd ed. Parkridge, IL: AAOS, 1992:355.)

quadriceps angle. Athletes who have generalized ligamentous laxity, increased femoral anteversion, or external tibial torsion are also predisposed to patellar instability.

Diagnosis

The athlete will complain of anteromedial knee pain, which can be confused with injuries to other medial structures such as the medial meniscus and collateral ligament. The knee will be swollen and tender along the medial patellar retinaculum. The patellar apprehension test should be positive. In this test, with the knee in full extension, laterally directed manual pressure is placed on the medial edge of the patella (Fig. 12.22). When the patient attempts to flex the knee, there is increasing pain, splinting, and a facial grimace that reflects appre-

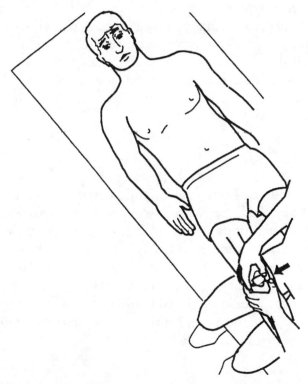

Figure 12.22 *The patella apprehension test for patellar instability. The examiner places laterally directed pressure on the patella with the knee extended. The initiation of knee flexion will then cause the patient to be apprehensive if the patella is unstable.* (Reproduced by permission from Gross J, Fetto J, Rosen E. Musculoskeletal examination. Cambridge, MA: Blackwell Science, 1995.)

hension. Tangential patellar radiographs may demonstrate abnormal patellar tilt or fractures of the lateral femoral groove or the medial patellar margin.

Treatment

The treatment is usually nonsurgical, especially for the first dislocation. Acutely the knee is treated with ice, compression, and splinting in full extension. Nonoperative management requires immobilization in full extension to facilitate healing of the medial patellar retinaculum. Full motion is permitted after 4 to 6 weeks. Rehabilitation focuses on restoration of quadriceps strength, particularly the vastus medialis. A neoprene sleeve with an anterior cutout and lateral patellar pad can be helpful. If the injury causes an osteochondral fracture of the patella or femoral groove, arthroscopic evaluation and treatment are warranted.

Surgical reconstruction may be necessary with recurrent patellar instability. Soft tissue procedures, such as a lateral patella retinaculum release with medial retinacular reefing, are preferred in children with open epiphyseal growth. In adults these procedures may be combined with an osteotomy and realignment of the tibial tuberosity.

Extensor Mechanism Disruption

The extensor mechanism of the knee comprises the quadriceps muscle and tendon, the bony patella, and the patellar tendon, which inserts upon the tibial tuberosity. Disruption of the extensor mechanism is seen in weight lifters and in older, unconditioned athletes. The mechanism involves a sudden forcible contraction of the quadriceps muscle causing rupture, usually at the tendon-bone junction. The tendon avulsion occurs at one of three sites, namely, the inferior or superior poles of the patella or occasionally the tibial tuberosity. The athlete will state that the knee "buckled" and may have difficulty arising from a seated position or ascending stairs.

Diagnosis

The knee is often held in a flexed position. The patient may place a hand on the anterior aspect of the knee when walking up an incline or rising from a chair. The integrity of the entire extensor mechanism of the knee is easily tested by asking the patient to perform a straight-leg raise. If the patient is unable to fully extend the knee, some element of the extensor mechanism is disrupted. A palpable gap or point tender-ness will help localize the site of injury.

A lateral flexed-knee x-ray can demonstrate proximal migration of the patella when disruption has occurred within the patellar tendon. If the distance from patella to tibial tuberosity is normal, the injury is most likely localized to the quadriceps tendon. A fracture of the patella is easily ruled out on a lateral knee radiograph. MRI scans and ultrasonography can be used to distinguish partial from total extensor tendon ruptures.

Treatment

Treatment is by direct surgical repair of the extensor mechanism. Nonoperative treatment is usually associated with marked quadriceps weakness and should be avoided.

Pediatric Knee Injuries

The bones of children are unique because they include a zone of growth cartilage, called the physis or growth plate, that adds length to growing long bones. These growth centers disappear and fuse in adulthood. The two most active growth zones in a child are those of the distal femur and the proximal tibia. Physeal cartilage is structur-ally weaker than ligament, collagen, or bone mineral. Therefore it is more likely for an immature athlete to sustain a growth plate injury than a ligament injury.

Diagnosis

The physical findings of a growth plate fracture are often indistin-guishable from those of ligament injuries. Yet one should always be suspicious that a joint injury in a child is actually a growth plate fracture. Stress radiographs (Fig. 12.23) make the distinction, as the stress on a growth plate fracture will result in widening of cartilagi-nous physis but not of the joint space as occurs with a pure ligament injury.

Treatment

These injuries require cast immobilization to protect the limb while the fracture heals. Displaced growth plate injuries often require surgi-cal reduction and fixation to secure proper fracture alignment. Total or partial irreversible growth plate cartilage damage can complicate growth plate fractures and result in either inequality of leg length or angular bony deformity, respectively. Long-term follow-up radio-

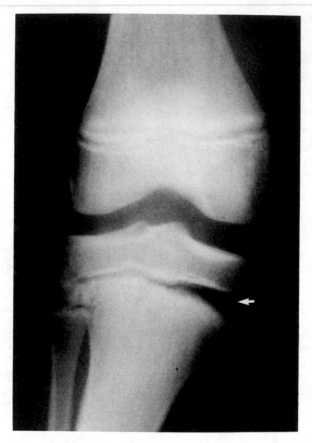

Figure 12.23 *What was thought to be a medial collateral ligament injury was a fracture of the tibial growth plate (arrow). Stress radiographs reveal widening of the medial tibial growth plate in a 10-year-old child.*

graphs are needed to document that the limb has continued to grow without deformity.

When evaluating a child or even an adult, it is extremely important to remember that knee pain may be referred. The obturator nerve primarily innervates the hip abductor muscles but also sends a sensory branch to the medial aspect of the knee. Consequently, hip pathology may manifest as a medial knee complaint. A hip examination should be part of every knee evaluation. Hip diagnoses that are frequently missed by a narrow focus upon the knee are stress fractures of the femoral neck in adults, slipped capital femoral epiphysis in children, and hip tumors in all age groups.

Most hip disorders can be detected by simply observing the patient's gait or by checking the range of motion of both hips. Hip pain causes a characteristic Trendelenburg limp in which the patient's trunk lurches over the affected hip during weight transference. The

Trendelenburg's lurch is due to hip abductor muscle weakness or pain or both. Manual muscle testing of the hip abductors will also cause pain and weakness. Comparison of passive hip motion to that of the unaffected side often demonstrates asymmetric and restricted motion.

Chronic Soft Tissue Knee Injuries

Chronic injuries occur in a noncontact mode from repetitive stress and overuse. They often result from training errors, when the athlete is pushed beyond a judicious amount of fatigue. Chronic injuries usually have a slow and insidious onset. Others may be associated with a specific injurious activity or event, yet the athlete is often able to continue participation, albeit at a lower level of performance.

All exercise is, in reality, the controlled application of traumatic stress to the collagenous tissues (muscle, ligament, tendon, and bone) of the body in such a way as to cause an increase in tissue bulk and strength. Inflammation is the body's natural healing response to injury from excessive stress. The reparative phases of the inflammatory process allow for the tissue to heal. Often this process results in a stronger structure that will be able to withstand similar amounts of stress in the future. When the amount of exercise-induced tissue trauma overwhelms the tissue's reparative capabilities, the inflammatory cycle remains thwarted in the earlier degradative stages and an overuse injury ensues. Thus the mainstay treatment for chronic inflammatory conditions is relative rest that protects the injured part and allows it to progress through the entire healing process (see Chapters 3 and 4 for further information). The following sections will describe the most common overuse injuries in and around the knee.

Tendinitis

Patellar Tendinitis

Patellar tendinitis results from repetitive stress and microscopic injury to the patellar tendon and occurs predominantly with jumping sports; therefore it is often called "jumper's knee." The diagnosis is often easily made. The athlete is tender anteriorly over the patellar tendon, which may be palpably swollen. The maximum tenderness is invariably at the patellar attachment site of the tendon near the inferior pole of the patella. Manually resisted quadriceps contraction with the knee placed in varying degrees of flexion may reproduce the athlete's discomfort. In contrast to ruptures of the quadriceps mechanism, the patient should be able to fully extend the knee against gravity. There should be no extension lag.

The treatment is based on relative rest. Heat and nonsteroidal anti-inflammatory medication are other helpful analgesic measures. Squatting, jumping, and stair climbing should be curtailed. The quadriceps muscle mass is maintained with isometric exercise and light eccentric strengthening. Quadriceps and hamstring muscle stretching exercises are also emphasized. Friction massage can also be helpful (see Chapter 5).

Quadriceps Tendinitis

Quadriceps tendinitis is similar to patellar tendinitis except that the site of tenderness is at the superior pole of the patella. This is the attachment site of the quadriceps tendon.

Iliotibial Tract Friction Syndrome

Iliotibial tract friction syndrome is a common cause of lateral knee pain in runners, especially if they are bowlegged or use shoes that are worn out on the lateral sole. The iliotibial tract originates from the pelvis and is composed of the fascial investment of the tensor fascia lata and gluteus maximus muscles (Fig. 12.24). At the knee it divides into an anterior segment, which is attached to the patella and guides patellar tracking. The posterior segment inserts on a special anterior (Gerdy's) tubercle of the tibia (see Fig. 12.8). As the knee flexes and extends, the iliotibial tract repeatedly crosses over the prominent lateral femoral epicondyle. Friction between tract and bone may cause either a bursitis or inflammation of the tract itself. Athletes with the syndrome complain of activity-related lateral knee pain that occurs several miles into a run.

The diagnosis can be made by palpation, which will disclose an area of tenderness over the distal iliotibial tract between Gerdy's tubercle and the lateral femoral epicondyle. The iliotibial tract may be tight and painful when subjected to Ober's test. To perform this test, the athlete is placed on his or her side with the normal leg down. Thigh adduction may be decreased or painful. With the thigh maximally adducted, symptoms are exacerbated by knee extension and lessened by flexion as the former places the iliotibial band under greater degrees of tension.

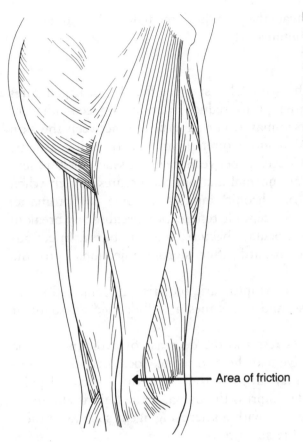

Figure 12.24 *The iliotibial tract moves over the lateral femoral epicondyle during knee motion. Friction between these two structures can cause a bursitis or inflammation of the tract itself.* (Redrawn by permission from Hughston JC, Walsh WM, Paddu G. Patella subluxation and dislocation. Philadelphia: WB Saunders, 1984:4.)

Area of friction

Popliteus Tendinitis

This form of tendinitis may be responsible for posterolateral knee pain associated with downhill running. The athlete will point to an area of tenderness that is just anterior to the femoral origin of the lateral collateral ligament, at the site of the popliteus tendon insertion. This muscle resists external rotation of the tibia and holds the femur posteriorly. The popliteus is stressed particularly with downhill running, as it resists anterior displacement of the femur and tibial rotation.

Hamstring Tendinitis

Hamstring tendinitis causes chronic posterior knee pain. The athlete will be discretely tender either over the medial hamstring tendons (semitendinosus, gracilis, and semimembranosus) or laterally over the biceps femoris tendon. Resisted hamstring muscle contraction (knee joint flexion) may aggravate the pain. Both medial and lateral tendons are rarely involved simultaneously.

Bursitis

A bursa is a sac lined by synovial tissue (see Fig. 12.5). It generates synovial fluid in an attempt to reduce friction between adjacent moving structures. Bursae may occur superficially between the skin and bone, or skin and tendon, often from poorly fitting athletic equipment. Bursae also develop between deeper tissues such as tendon and bone. Bursae are normal anatomic structures, which when aggravated by acute or chronic injuries become symptomatic. Subcutaneous bursae are susceptible to infection because any break in the overlying skin may inoculate bacteria into the bursa. Infectious bursitis is a particular hazard after steroid injections into the bursa.

Physical examination of symptomatic bursitis will demonstrate an area of point tenderness, and sometimes a well-defined fluctuant or crepitant swelling.

The treatment involves rest and the decrease or avoidance of the inciting activity. Protective pads help to reduce local irritation. Nonsteroidal anti-inflammatory drugs can alleviate the associated pain. Needle aspiration can decompress the bursa. If the fluid is cloudy, it should be cultured. Injection with a sclerosing agent such as tetracycline may prevent bursal recurrence.

Prepatellar Bursitis

The prepatellar bursa exists between the dermis and the skin overlying the patella (see Fig. 12.5). It is seen in sports requiring kneeling such as surfing and wrestling.

Pes Anserine Bursitis

The pes anserine bursa lies between the medial hamstring tendons (sartorius, gracilis, and semitendinosus) and the proximal medial tibia (see Fig. 12.5). The pes anserine bursa is inferior to the joint line, which helps to distinguish it from medial joint line tenderness due to meniscal injury.

Voshell's Bursitis

Voshell's bursa is located between the medial collateral ligament and the tibia and can be seen in athletes who have increased valgus knee alignment. The findings of an inflamed Voshell's bursa are similar to those of pes anserine bursitis. However, discomfort from this bursa should not be associated with hamstring muscle function.

Synovitis

The knee joint is a snovium-lined cavity with a large suprapatellar pouch (see Fig. 12.5). The lining contains synovial cells that remove particulate debris and secrete joint fluid to lubricate the moving joint surfaces. Synovial fluid also contains the nutrients that sustain joint surface hyaline cartilage cells. Inflammation of this joint-lining tissue (synovitis) can occur after an acute or chronic trauma to the knee. Inflamed, hypertrophic synovial tissue also is a feature of inflammation disorders such as rheumatoid arthritis or systemic lupus erythematosus. Rheumatologic diseases usually affect several joints simultaneously. Painful synovitis is also seen in Lyme disease, which is caused by an infectious spirochete introduced by tick bites. Lyme disease should be considered when the sporting activity occurs outdoors in endemic environments.

Popliteal (Baker's) Cyst

A Baker's cyst represents ballooning of the synovium-lined joint capsule. It typically exits the knee between the medial head of the gastrocnemius and the semimembranosus muscles. Although fluid-filled, a popliteal cyst is not a bursa but rather a secondary manifestation of any condition that causes chronic inflammation of the knee, such as a meniscus tear, intra-articular loose body, or knee synovitis. When a popliteal cyst ruptures, joint fluid can dissect into the calf can cause massive leg swelling and pain.

The diagnosis of a popliteal cyst can be made by direct palpation of the mass. Arthrography or an MRI scan will verify the diagnosis and demonstrate its communication with the joint cavity. The cyst usually resolves after correction of the intra-articular pathology. Bakers cysts occur mainly on the posteromedial knee. A posterolateral knee mass should raise the suspicion of tumor. The symptoms of a ruptured Baker's cyst mimic venous thrombosis of the calf. A venous Doppler ultrasound examination will help rule out deep vein thrombosis.

Medial Synovial Plica (Shelf)

The medial plica is a focal synovial thickening interposed between the patella and femoral condyle (see Fig. 12.6). Twenty percent of all knees have a vestigial fold of synovium that is a remnant of tissue that did not fully resorb when knee joint cavitation occurred during embryonic development. Some plicae may also arise from direct synovial irritation. In some athletes this fold can become painful from chronic irritation.

The symptoms are anterior in location and similar to those of patellofemoral overload. The athlete will complain of anteromedial knee pain that is aggravated by activities requiring flexion. There may be patellar clicking or actual catching with knee joint motion. If thickened and swollen, the plica may be directly palpable and tender. If synovial hypertrophy is diffuse and other joints are involved, a rheumatologic cause should be sought.

Many plicae respond to the same nonoperative treatment program described for patellofemoral overload. Only those recalcitrant to conservative measures require arthroscopic resection.

Patellofemoral Overload (Chondromalacia Patella)

Anterior knee pain has often been ascribed to early cartilage degeneration and, thus, dubbed chondromalacia from the Latin root *chondro* for cartilage, and *malacia*, softening. It is a common knee problem and is usually secondary to subtle patellar tracking abnormalities. During normal knee flexion and extension, the patella tracks in an anterior groove between the femoral condyles (see Fig. 12.1). Many factors act to keep the patella centralized in this groove including the wall height of the femoral condyles, balance between the vastus medialis and vastus lateralis muscles, as well as the support of the patellar retinacula and the iliotibial band (Fig. 12.25). The mild form of joint surface arthritis implied by the term chondromalacia is not always observed surgically and is probably a misnomer.

Patellofemoral overload occurs when patellar tracking becomes unbalanced. This can occur from tightness of the lateral patellar retinaculum or iliotibial band; weakness of the vastus medialis; an increased quadriceps (Q) angle associated with genu valgum (knocked knees), or in-toeing from femoral anteversion. Ligamentous laxity and an elongated patella tendon are also associated with patellar instability. Women are predisposed to patellofemoral problems because their broader pelvic structure increases their Q angle (see Fig. 12.21).

Patellofemoral pain is typically anterior in location. It is intensified by activities that load the knee in flexion and subject the patella to high compression forces. Such activities include squatting, kneeling,

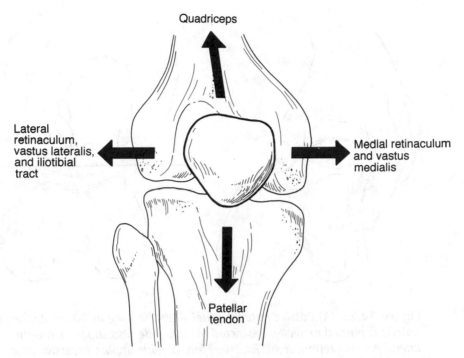

Quadriceps

Lateral
retinaculum,
vastus lateralis,
and iliotibial
tract

Medial retinaculum
and vastus
medialis

Patellar
tendon

Figure 12.25 *The patella tracks in the femoral groove and is balanced by opposing structures.* (Redrawn by permission from Fulkerson FP, Hungerford DS. Disorders of the patellofemoral joint, 2nd ed. Baltimore: Williams and Wilkins, 1990:14.)

rising from a chair, prolonged sitting, and ascending or descending stairs and hills.

Physical examination often reveals palpable patellofemoral crepitation during knee motion. Crepitation per se is often a normal finding. It is only of concern when associated with symptoms such as pain or swelling. Simple gait observation may reveal a genu valgum habitus or in-toeing from increased femoral anteversion. The medial patellar facet may be painful on palpation. Pain may be produced by passive compression of the patella into the femur. A better-tolerated test is to place the knee in 120° of flexion and have the patient extend the knee against resistance. This condition, which loads the patella, can reproduce the patient's pain.

Tightness of the patellar retinacula can be assessed by the patellar glide test (Fig. 12.26). The knee is flexed 30° and the patella is passively translated medially and laterally. The patella is divided into quadrants. Passive glide greater than three quadrants laterally suggests that there is excessive medial retinacular laxity. Less than one

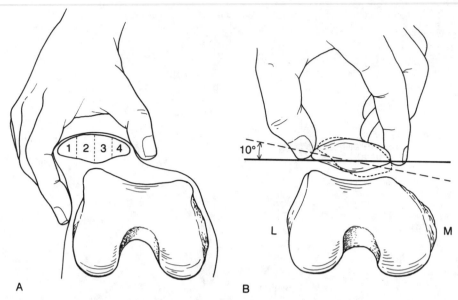

Figure 12.26 *(A) Passive patellar glide. With the knee in 30° of flexion, the patella is pushed medially. Restricted medial glide also suggests a tight lateral patellar retinaculum. Excessive lateral glide implies excessive medial retinacular laxity.* (Redrawn by permission from Chapman MW. Operative orthopedics, 2nd ed. Philadelphia: JB Lippincott, 1993:2413.) *(B) The patellar tilt test. With the knee flexed 10° the lateral patella is tilted anteriorly. Decreased tilt is seen with a tight lateral patellar retinaculum.* (Redrawn by permission from Fu F, Mayday, M. Arthroscopic lateral release and the lateral patter syndrome. Orthopaedic Clinics 1992;23:603.)

quadrant of medial laxity implies a tight lateral retinaculum. The patellar tilt test is done with the knee in extension. Lack of passive lateral tilt is consistent with a tight lateral retinaculum.

The treatment involves rest, heat, the use of anti-inflammatory medication, and the avoidance of aggravating activities. The use of progressive resistance exercises over a full arc of knee motion actually increases patellofemoral contact pressures and aggravates this condition. Squats, leg presses, and in particular quadriceps extension exercises in an open chain manner over a full arc of motion are to be avoided. Emphasis is placed on isometric quadriceps-strengthening exercises such as straight-leg raising. Quadriceps, hamstring, and iliotibial band stretching exercises are critical to successful management of patellofemoral problems. Patients with a tight lateral retinaculum or lateral subluxation that is resistant to therapy, may require surgical treatment such as a lateral retinacular release.

Conditions that must be excluded in the differential diagnosis of patellofemoral overload are patellar instability and osteochondritis dissecans of the medial femoral condyle or the patella itself. X-rays can help to identify these conditions.

Osgood-Schlatter Disease (Tibial Tubercle Apophysitis)

The patellar tendon inserts upon the tibial tuberosity, which has a growth plate or apophysis. In very athletic and often overweight children, excessive quadriceps tension can cause microscopic injury to the tibial tubercle growth plate.

The child will be swollen and tender over the patellar tendon insertion on the anterior tibia. Hyperflexion of the knee, squatting, and resisted quadriceps contraction will reproduce the pain. X-rays may show fragmentation of the tibial tubercle apophysis.

The treatment may require immobilization in full knee extension. Quadriceps stretching is an important part of the maintenance program once symptoms subside. The symptoms will disappear permanently once the growth plates close at the end of growth.

Sindig-Larsen-Johansson Disease

Similar to Osgood-Schlatter disease, Sindig-Larsen-Johansson disease involves the distal patellar pole. This is the pediatric version of a jumper's knee and is due to repetitive microtrauma. The treatment protocol is identical to that of Osgood-Schlatter disease.

Differential Diagnosis of Knee Pain in Athletes

Anterior Knee Pain

Acute Pain

- ✘ Patellar instability
- ✘ Extensor mechanism injury
- ✘ Patella fracture
- ✘ Growth plate fracture
- ✘ Hip fracture

Chronic Pain

- ✘ Patellofemoral overload (chondromalacia patella)
- ✘ Recurrent patellar instability
- ✘ Patellar tendinitis (jumper's knee)

✘ Prepatellar bursitis
✘ Osgood-Schlatter disease
✘ Sindig-Larsen-Johansson disease
✘ Medial synovial plica
✘ Osteochondritis dissecans
✘ Hip pathology (e.g., tumor)

Medial Knee Pain

Acute Pain

✘ Medial cruciate ligament injury
✘ Medial meniscus tear
✘ Patellar instability
✘ Growth plate fracture
✘ Hip fracture

Chronic Pain

✘ Meniscal injury
✘ Medial synovial plica
✘ Pes anserine or Voshell's bursitis
✘ Tibial plateau stress fracture
✘ Hip pathology

Lateral Knee Pain

Acute Pain

✘ Lateral cruciate ligament injury
✘ Lateral meniscus tear
✘ Lateral tibial plateau fracture (older patient)

Chronic Pain

✘ Iliotibial band friction syndrome
✘ Proximal tibiofibular joint instability
✘ Popliteus tendinitis
✘ Discoid meniscus

Differential Diagnosis of Common Knee Symptoms

Giving Way

✘ Meniscus tear
✘ Anterior cruciate ligament injury

✘ Patellar instability
✘ Loose body

Locking

✘ Meniscal tear, displaced
✘ Loose body

Hemarthrosis

✘ Anterior cruciate ligament tear
✘ Meniscus tear
✘ Fracture
✘ Patellar dislocation
✘ Synovial contusion

Suggested Readings

American Academy of Orthopaedic Surgeons. Athletic training and sports medicine. 2nd ed. Parkridge, IL: American Academy of Orthopaedic Surgeons, 1991.

Brody PM. Running injuries, prevention and management. CIBA Symp 1987;39(3).

Feagin JA Jr, ed. The crucial ligaments: diagnosis and treatment of ligamentous injuries about the knee. New York: Churchill Livingstone, 1994.

Fulkerson JP, Hungerford DS. Disorders of the patellofemoral joint. 2nd ed. Baltimore: Williams & Wilkins, 1990.

Insall JN, Windsor RE, Scott WN, et al, eds. Surgery of the knee. 2nd ed. New York: Churchill Livingstone, 1993.

Mow VC, Arnoczky SP, Jackson DW, eds. Knee meniscus; basic and clinical foundations. New York: Raven Press, 1992.

Netter FH. Musculoskeletal system: Part III. Trauma, evaluation and management. The CIBA collection of medical illustrations. Summit, NJ: CIBA, 1993.

Schenck RC, Heckman JD. Injuries of the knee. CIBA Symp 1993;45(1).

CHAPTER 13

Lower Leg Injuries

Uffe Jørgensen

The lower leg can be involved in 5% to 15% of all injuries in certain sports. In particular, running and jumping sports are associated with more lower leg injuries. Normally, lower leg injuries have a good prognosis. However, they often become chronic if not treated correctly.

Lower leg injuries can be divided into acute or chronic injuries. There is usually no doubt about the etiology of acute injuries. A jump, kick, fall, or collision can clearly mark the onset of the injury. However, occasionally some predisposing factors can be involved, which have to be addressed in order to avoid reinjury. Typical acute injuries are muscle strains or contusions. More rarely tendon ruptures are seen, such as those involving the Achilles tendon. Chronic injuries are more insidious in their onset. The offending activity is not always immediately obvious. Common causes are sudden changes in training regimens, inadequate equipment, and faulty techniques. In addition to these external factors, there may be predisposing internal factors such as inflexibility and weakness. This chapter will discuss common acute and chronic injuries of the lower leg between the knee and ankle.

Muscle Strain

An acute muscle strain is a sudden tear in the muscle-tendon unit (see Chapters 2, 3, and 4 for general information). Most acute muscle strains are described by the patient as a sudden pain, usually in the posterior part of the lower leg. Some patients will describe that they felt a string snap and subsequently experienced a hot feeling in the injured area. In severe muscle strains the function of the muscle is impaired immediately and the athlete is unable to continue. Smaller strains, after a period of rest, allow the athlete to continue sports activities. However, when the athlete wakes up the next morning, a swollen lower leg, pain, and a loss of function become obvious.

The mechanism of muscle strains is similar to that of strains elsewhere in the body (see Chapter 2). Tired muscles and muscles that are not flexible enough may be predisposed to injury. Therefore prevention and rehabilitation of these injuries include endurance and strength training as well as constant attention to their flexibility through stretching exercises.

In theory, any muscle of the lower leg can sustain a strain. The posterior muscles, however, account for the vast majority of these injuries. In particular, the gastrocnemius muscle is susceptible to this injury, and the injury is often called "tennis leg." Physical findings are usually limited to localized tenderness and pain when using the muscle. Complete, grade III ruptures are unusual in this area. Non-steroidal anti-inflammatory drugs can be helpful in controlling the pain and swelling.

Treatment

The acute treatment is with rest, ice, compression, and elevation (the RICE principle; see Chapter 5). Mobilization is begun as soon as possible to regain the range of motion and avoid scar tissue formation. It is somewhat controversial when exactly one should start to stretch a muscle that has recently been strained. However, a recommended treatment is to regain range of motion as soon as the pain allows and to use the muscle within the limits of comfort. A little pain is to be expected, but when the pain becomes severe, the athlete should stop. This is a commonly accepted guideline for both stretching and strengthening of the injured muscle. For instance, the athlete with a moderate to severe strain should not focus on vigorous stretching for the first week. After this initial peroid of rest, the flexibility training is started gradually in order to regain excursion of the muscle. In general, athletes should not stretch through severe pain as it may worsen the strain. Ultrasound is often used during the healing phases of a muscle strain to promote the proliferative and maturation response.

Tennis Leg

Injury to the back side of the leg at the muscle-tendon junction or medial head of the gastrocnemius is called a tennis leg (Fig. 13.1). It happens suddenly and can be misdiagnosed as an Achilles tendon rupture. As opposed to Achilles tendon ruptures, there is a tender area and sometimes a palpable defect in the muscle belly itself. This can be near the origin from the femur or close to the junction with the Achilles tendon. The injury is usually a partial tear (grade I or II) and does not require absolute immobilization. Early light stretching is recommended, but one should be careful in the beginning not to worsen the injury. Once the pain has subsided, the treatment also includes strengthening of the muscle usually by toe-raising exercises. Sport-specific exercises and return to sports can start 4 to 8 weeks following the injury.

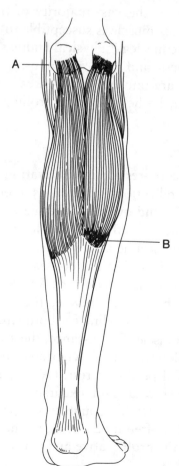

Figure 13.1 *Tennis leg is a rupture of the calf muscle at the origin near the femoral attachment (A) or at the muscle-tendon junction (B).*

Muscle Contusion

Muscle contusions are acute injuries often caused by kicks of opponents in collision sports. The contusion causes bleeding and swelling in the muscle, and this impairs the muscle function. The use of the muscle is also inhibited because of pain.

Differential diagnosis includes fractures of the fibula, where function of the muscle surrounding the fractures is also inhibited because of pain. More serious are the fractures of tibia or of both tibia and fibula. Combined fracture of tibia and fibula results in a complete loss of stability and function. Patients with these fractures should be referred to a specialist for further diagnosis and treatment.

Treatment

The RICE principle (see Chapter 5) is applied in order to stop the bleeding and decrease the swelling and pain. If one can diminish the bleeding immediately, the rehabilitation can be started earlier. Commonly ice is applied for 15 to 20 minutes two to three times a day or more in the first week or two. At the same time muscle exercises are started. First, range-of-motion exercises are used. If the muscle can move the surrounding joints through a normal range of motion, it will heal relatively fast. These minor contusions often allow continued activity and may be resolved in 2 to 3 weeks. However, severe contusions with markedly diminished function may take 6 to 8 weeks or more to recover. It is essential to regain the range of motion and strength in these muscles before the athlete returns to sports. As for muscle strains, nonsteroidal anti-inflammatory drugs and ultrasound are often used to decrease inflammation and promote healing.

Myositis Ossificans

After a muscle contusion myositis ossificans can develop as a complication. Myositis ossificans is bone formation in an area of injured muscle tissue. The area becomes hard, and the ossification can be seen on x-ray. Adequate rest will usually calm down the process, and surgical removal is rarely needed (see Chapter 11 for more information).

Acute Compartment Syndrome

Another complication of a severe muscle contusion is acute compartment syndrome, which can have dramatic consequences. Compartment syndrome develops when arterial bleeding caused by the injury increases pressure within the muscle fascia. When the pressure exceeds the outflow pressure in the venous system (Fig. 13.2), compartment syndrome can develop. Lack of oxygen and nutrients affects the muscles, and if this condition is not reversed, the muscle tissue within the compartment will suffer permanent damage. Symptoms of the acute compartment syndrome are (1) pain with use of the muscle, (2) swelling and relative tightness of the injured compartment compared with the opposite leg, and (3) pain in the compartment if the muscles within the compartment are passively stretched (for instance, pushing the toes and foot in a plantar direction in anterior compartment syndrome).

If two or three signs are present, the patient should be referred to an appropriate facility for possible surgical treatment. The patient should be evaluated with invasive pressure measurements.

Other signs such as absence of distal pulses and decreased sensibility are late findings, and permanent muscle injury may have occurred already. Therefore one should always think of the possibility of an

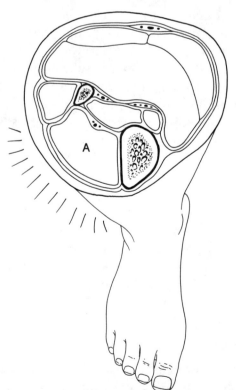

Figure 13.2 *The fascial compartments of the lower leg. Compartment syndrome is particularly common in the anterior compartment (A).*

acute compartment syndrome developing. Prevention may be possible by immediate application of the RICE principle. When it is invasively confirmed, acute compartment syndrome is treated by surgical fasciotomy, which opens the muscular fascia in order to decrease the pressure in the area.

Achilles Tendon Ruptures

The Achilles tendon is the most frequently ruptured tendon in the lower leg. It is also one of the slowest-healing acute injuries, as the time from rupture to full function often is 3 to 9 months depending on the activity level.

Mechanism of Injury

Often Achilles tendon ruptures occur in sports like basketball, tennis, volleyball, badminton, and other sports in which sudden stops and jumps are performed. Many patients with Achilles tendon ruptures have had previous Achilles tendinitis or peritendinitis. The rupture occurs when the patient is landing on the foot, trying to absorb the energy by eccentric action of the gastocnemius-soleus muscle. The rupture typically occurs 3 to 4 cm above the tendon insertion into the calcaneus.

Symptoms and Findings

These patients complain of immediate pain but often do not immediately notice the loss of function of the muscle. Other intact muscles often continue to allow them to walk normally. The complete rupture can be diagnosed when one squeezes the gastrocnemius-soleus muscle belly and the foot does not move in plantar flexion (Thomson's test) (Fig. 13.3). Typically a defect is seen or felt at the site of the rupture.

Treatment

The treatment of Achilles tendon ruptures is controversial. However, many feel that in active athletes the treatment of choice is surgical repair of the ruptured tendon. This results in a lower risk of rerupture and improved function compared with treatment by cast immobilization.

Rehabilitation

Often a brace is used for 3 to 8 weeks after repair of the ruptured Achilles tendon. Newer studies are adding range-of-motion exercise

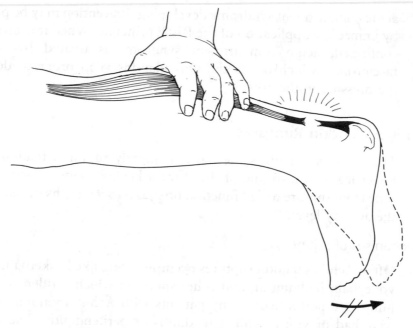

Figure 13.3 *Thomson's test is positive for Achilles tendon rupture if compression of the calf does not result in planter flexion of the foot.*

as early as 1 week after the repair to stimulate the tendon and keep the muscles in as good shape as possible. Once the tendon is healed, typically after 6 to 8 weeks, mobilization is started. Initially a heel lift of 1 to 2 cm is recommended in order to unload the tendon. Subsequently a strengthening exercise program of the gastrocnemius-soleus muscle is recommended within the limits of pain. Strengthening is usually started by toe-raising exercises.

The principle is for the athlete to regain range of motion, strength, and finally endurance of the Achilles tendon complex before returning to sports. Within the first 3 months it is recommended to avoid jumping and running up stairs on the toes because this puts a tremendous load on the Achilles tendon. The tendon may not regain its final strength for as long as 1 to 2 years after the injury. Therefore sports activities with high speed and high forces are often delayed for several months. Return at 6 months is more reasonable in some athletes to avoid reruptures.

Other Tendon Ruptures

The plantaris longus is a small, insignificant muscle next to the gastrocnemius muscle that reportedly can rupture. It can simulate other muscle strains. However, the prognosis is much better, as the athlete can often return to full activities in 1 or 2 weeks because the gastrocnemius compensates for its function. Tendons from the tibialis anterior and posterior and the peroneal tendons can rupture. However, the symptoms of those ruptures are typically around the ankle and are beyond the scope of this chapter.

Overuse Injuries

Overuse injuries are most frequent in endurance sports, such as long distance running, cycling, and swimming. In long distance running approximately 25% of the injuries are localized to the knee, 11% around the Achilles tendon, and 7% to the plantar fascia of the foot. About 10% of the overuse injuries occur in the shin area (shin splints), which includes periostitis, stress fractures, and chronic compartment syndrome.

The mechanism of injury in overuse problems is discussed in more detail in Chapter 2. In general, the repetitive stress of the sport can cause a gradual injury in the weakest part of the involved extremity. When the repetitive stress is present for a long duration, virtually every athlete will eventually sustain an overuse injury in some structures in the lower leg (Fig. 13.4). The risk of injury is even higher if there is some degree of malalignment or if there are structures in the lower extremity that have not been rehabilitated adequately after an injury. If the structures are inflexible or weak, an overuse syndrome is easily provoked. The potential factors involved with

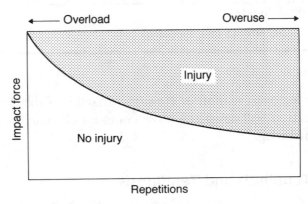

Figure 13.4 *The relation between impact forces, number of repetitions, and likelihood of lower leg injuries. As the forces or repetitions increase, the likelihood of injuries increases.*

Table 13.1   Overuse injury etiology

1. Training errors

Rapid changes in training: intensity or duration or both
Excessive training intensity or load
Return to exercise after a long break
Changes in running gait
A bad technique

2. Biomechanical malalignment

Excessive pronation
Forefoot varus or valgus
Hindfoot varus or valgus
Cavus foot
Flat foot
Tibia varum (genu varum)
Leg length differences
Soft heel pads (decreased shock absorption)
Ankle instability
Relative stiffness or decreased strength and endurance in the muscle-tendon
    complex

3. Shoe design

Low shock absorption
Soft heel counter (that does not support the heel)
Wrong shoe type with respect to running type (neutral runner, supinator,
    pronator)

4. Surface

Hard surfaces
Sudden shift of surfaces

5. Medical diseases

Inflammatory arthritis (enthesopathy)

lower leg overuse injuries are summarized in Table 13.1. The following section will cover the most common chronic overuse injuries of the lower leg.

Achilles Tendinitis and Tendinosis

Pain in or around the Achilles tendon is an extremely common overuse injury in the lower leg (Fig. 13.5). The problem can consist of inflammation around the tendon, which is often called tendinitis,

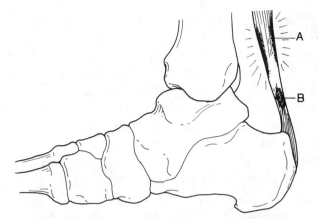

Figure 13.5 *Achilles tendon pain can be caused by inflammation in the peritendineum (peritendinitis) (A) or in the tendon (tendinitis) (B), or both.*

paratenonitis, or peritendinitis. In these cases the sheath around the Achilles tendon is inflammed and swollen.

Another form of an Achilles tendon problem is tendinosis, in which the tendon itself is the focus of injury. This involves a degeneration of the tendon tissue. It is possible that this is made possible by aging of the tendon as this problem is more frequently seen in athletes over 30 years of age. Combinations of peritendinitis and tendinosis are also often seen.

Symptoms and Findings

Pain in the tendon typically starts when the athlete begins to exercise. It often disappears after the warm-up. The pain often recurs after the sports activity. In addition, the tendon will feel stiff the next morning. More severe tendon problems may result in continuous, chronic pain anytime the tendon is stressed including walking and standing.

The diagnosis of an Achilles tendon problem is made by palpation of the tendon. In typical paratenonitis or peritendinitis, the sheath will be swollen in the acute phase. There will be redness over a greater area, and often crepitus can be felt when the tendon moves. In more chronic cases, there can be some irregularities or nodules with palpation along the tendon.

The pain in tendinosis can be at the point approximately 2 inches or 5 cm from the distal insertion of the tendon into the calcaneus. There can also be swelling and pain directly over the insertion into the calcaneus. In chronic cases there is often thickening of the tendon at those sites. In patients who developed the injury following a sudden jump or stop, there can be pain directly at the insertion site between the calcaneus and the tendon, owing to a partial rupture in that area.

Ultrasonography or magnetic resonance imaging (MRI) scans can visualize partial ruptures in the tendon.

The mechanism of injury to some degree involves repetitive over-use. The development of the injury is directly associated with the function of the tendon. During the running motion the tendon will be tight at heel strike and absorb part of the shock at landing by vibrating as a violin string. In the next phase of the running motion, the foot moves into pronation ("flat-footed" position), which brings the calcaneus from a varus position at heel strike to a valgus position. This causes a sideward movement of the Achilles tendon. During the subsequent push-off phase, the whole process is reversed. The gastrocnemius-soleus muscle pulls the Achilles tendon and the calcaneus in the reverse direction. The large vibrations and movements can explain the development of an inflammation.

Predisposing factors can greatly increase the risk of developing Achilles tendon problems. If the tendon is relatively weak or tight, it will be less resistant to this constant loading. In athletes using running shoes with low or no shock absorption or with a thin heel pad that has low shock-absorbing capacity, the vibrations at heel strike will increase accordingly. Athletes with high arches (cavus foot) have a decreased shock absorption capacity in the foot and a tighter Achilles tendon. They are also at increased risk because of their stiff feet. Conversely, athletes with flat feet have the problem of hyperpronation with instability in the hind foot. This increases the sideways movement of the tendon, and thereby the load.

Tendon sheath inflammation and bursitis around the Achilles tendon are most often caused by irritation of the shoe. A stiff heel counter produces friction between the shoe and the tendon sheath, and subsequently an inflammation can develop. If this occurs chronically, a problem can develop with a bunion-like process on the back of the calcaneus. The bone is produced in response to the constant irritation. These "pump bumps" can be most irritating for a runner and may need to be surgically removed. It is important to remember that patients with gout and inflammatory arthritis such as rheumatoid arthritis and Reiter's syndrome can develop spontaneous peritendinitis and tendinitis.

Treatment

The treatment of Achilles tendon problems is primarily based on identifying the offending, etiologic factors. Often training errors are an important factor and need to be addressed. Intensity and duration of the exercise are decreased below the pain level. Increases thereafter are only small and made gradually to avoid recurrences. In addition, malalignment problems such as overpronation or low shock-absorbing capacity in the heel pad may have to be addressed. A custom-molded orthotic insert or the use of a shock-absorbing heel cup can benefit these patients (Fig. 13.6). A tight and weak Achilles tendon–gastrocnemius–soleus complex is placed on a stretching and strengthening program. This is particularly a problem in patients with chronic cases in whom there is a subconscious unloading of the injured leg.

In the more acute stage of peritendinitis, icing is recommended for 15 to 20 minutes several times a day. Nonsteroidal anti-inflammatory drugs can be helpful to control the pain and swelling. Once the swelling has subsided, the stretching and strengthening are started. The athlete can stretch the tendon until it feels sore, but should stop when it starts to become painful. This guideline is also used in the strength training. Strengthening is performed by toe-raising or squatting exercises standing on boths legs and gradually increasing the speed. Sets with 15 to 20 repetitions are used, and the load can be gradually increased with a barbell on the shoulders. Occasionally a heel lift of 1 to 2 cm can be helpful to avoid extreme stretch of the tendon during daily activities. If conservative treatment is not successful in 3 to 4 months, an orthopedic surgeon can be consulted to discuss the possibility of an operation to excise the diseased tendon tissue.

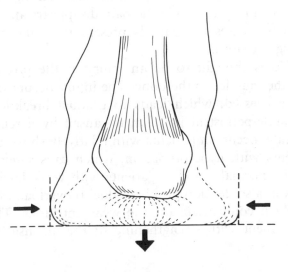

Figure 13.6 *A heel cup in the shoe can compress the heel pad and can increase the shock absorption at heel strike up to 50%. At the same time it provides stability of the hindfoot and thereby diminishes pronation.*

Prevention

Many Achilles tendon problems can be prevented by avoiding training errors. It is important to gradually build up a training program without too many sudden changes. The use of shock-absorbing, stable shoes also decreases the load. Good endurance, strength, and flexibility of the Achilles tendon–muscle complex decreases the possibility of injury. Only runners who have hyperpronation should use a shoe that compensates for this. If a runner with a physiologic amount of pronation uses a shoe that compensates for hyperpronation, the normal shock absorption capacity is actually decreased. This will increase the demands on the tendon and thereby provoke injuries.

Shin Splints

Chronic painful conditions localized on the shin area of the lower leg are called shin splints. They can be medial, lateral, or posterior to the tibia. The chronic pain of the lower leg typically can be caused by four different conditions: tibial periostitis, stress fracture, chronic compartment syndrome, or a small fascial muscle hernia in the muscular septum.

Tibial Periostitis

In traction periostitis the pain is found on the inner site of the tibia, typically the central one third of the tibia (Fig. 13.7). The tenderness in this area is aggravated by moving the fingers up and down the inner side of the tibia. Pain in this area develops in the late landing phase and push-off phase of running. Initially the pain disappears after the warm-up, but in severe cases the pain is present throughout the running and jumping activities.

Traction periostitis is thought to be an injury at the proximal attachment sites of the muscles to the bone. The injury occurs when the muscles are overstressed, which leads to gradual breakdown. Irritation of the muscle-periosteal junction is caused by a relative overload. This typically occurs in patients with relatively short, tight muscles or in patients with hyperpronation, which causes relative tightness in otherwise normal muscles. Patients with weak intrinsic muscles in the foot can also develop problems due to overload of the long toe flexors, which compensate for the weak intrinsics. These patients require treatment with strengthening of the intrinsic foot muscles.

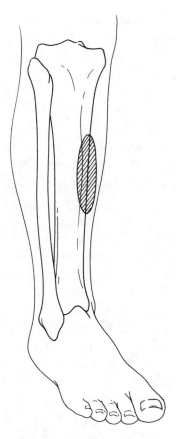

Figure 13.7 *Shin splint symptoms due to traction periostitis are typically felt along the medial edge of the tibia.*

Treatment

One has to first find the cause of the injury. If there is a predisposing condition such as hyperpronation, this should be compensated for by either a special shoe or insole. This can prevent the hyperpronation and stretch of the muscles involved. Athletes with weak intrinsic foot muscles often develop hammer toes and should have an intrinsic muscle-strengthening program.

In all patients, increased shock absorption in the shoe will decrease the initial impact on the muscle and therefore enable the patient to do more. In severe cases, when the condition is chronic and unresponsive, an operation can be an option. This involves stripping the periosteum and thereby releasing the tension within the muscles.

Stress Fracture

An important differential diagnosis in shin splints is a stress fracture. A stress fracture can be considered a fatigue fracture of the bone. A stress fracture can develop as the result of repeated, forceful muscle contractions around the bone causing small, repetitive bending loads on the bone. In addition, the bone reacts more slowly to the increasing load than the muscles do. The muscles get increasingly stronger but the bone cannot follow that same rate of increase. If the stress continues, a fracture can develop. The bone cannot rebuild and remodel fast enough before a new, higher load is put on it by the stronger muscles. Individual bone trabeculae collapse, causing "microfractures." This eventually accumulates into the so-called stress fracture. The stress fracture can vary from a minor partial fracture (stress reaction) to a complete fracture with even potential displacement of the bone fragments.

The symptoms start with a dull pain after exercise. Later the pain can increase until there is pain with every foot strike and eventually also when walking. The pain is concentrated in the injured area with local point tenderness. Eventually swelling can be seen. Compared with that of traction periostitis, the pain of a stress fracture is concentrated in a much smaller area, and there can be a distinct swelling in the area. Sometimes the diagnosis can be made with plain radiographs. A small crack can be visible, and later, during the healing phase, the healing bone (callus) can be seen. Small stress fractures can be difficult to see on plain radiographs. The diagnosis is confirmed by performing an isotope bone scan. Tibial periostitis will also show activity on a bone scan, but it is over a long, diffuse area of the bone surface that corresponds to the painful periosteum. On the other hand, a stress fracture extends across the bone and marrow in a very localized area, which results in a discrete hot spot on the bone scan. Depending on the severity of the fracure, this hot spot can extend all the way across the bone.

Treatment

Stress fractures in the lower leg, typically the tibia, can be treated by improving the patient's shock absorption through shock-absorbing running shoes or insoles. This allows more compression around the heel at heel strike in order to increase the shock absorption (increased compression around the heel pad can improve the shock absorption by 50%). Pain-provoking activity should be avoided, and for very active sports people running in water (aqua jogging) is an ideal way to maintain cardiovascular fitness. Bicycling is also a possibility because it avoids direct impact on the lower leg. Most stress fractures in the tibia or fibula can be treated in this fashion and will heal in 6 to 8 weeks. Occasionally, nonhealing stress fractures require casting or even surgical treatment if successive radiographs fail to show improvement.

Chronic Compartment Syndrome

The third condition leading to shin splint symptoms is chronic compartment syndrome. With increased exercise the muscle enlarges; however, sometimes the surrounding fascia cannot accommodate this enlargement. In addition, when the muscle exercises, the volume of blood entering the muscle increases, which also causes a temporary increase in the size of the muscle. If there is not enough space in the fascial compartment, the pressure will gradually increase, which in turn inhibits the outflow in the venous system. This causes further engorgement of the muscle and a greater increase in pressure, which eventually leads to slowing of the arterial inflow. Ischemia develops in the muscles, and this causes pain.

Patients with chronic compartment syndrome typically first notice pain after they have been exercising for a while. Runners often indicate that the pain comes after a predictable amount of running. Then they have to stop because of the severity of the pain, and after about 5 minutes of rest they can start running again.

With a typical history the diagnosis can often be made with high accuracy. However, tibia periostitis and stress fracture should be ruled out by palpating for tender areas along the tibia. If there is tenderness, one should remember that compartment syndrome can be seen in conjunction with stress fractures or, more typically, periostitis. The diagnosis can be confirmed by an invasive measurement of the pressure in the compartment at rest, during exercise, and immediately after exercise.

The most common chronic compartment syndrome in the lower extremity is on the outer (lateral) side of the tibia in the anterior compartment. The symptoms in anterior compartment syndrome are worsened by impact from landing when the tibialis anterior is active. Compartment syndromes can be seen, but less commonly, in the lateral (peroneal), deep posterior, and posterior compartments. Occasionally the chronic posterior compartment syndrome is preceded by a muscle rupture. Later, the athlete can develop a compartment syndrome from the formation of scar tissue in the compartment.

Treatment

The initial treatment in most athletes includes a decrease in the sports activities that precipitate the symptoms. Vigorous stretching of the involved muscles is recommended. Increased shock absorption with better running shoes or insoles is particularly helpful for those with anterior compartment problems. Avoidance of running on hard surfaces and downhill running also can diminish the symptoms. Once the symptoms have subsided, the sports activities should be increased again only gradually. Athletes who fail to respond and have documented increased pressure during and after exercise should consider a surgical fasciotomy. During this operation the fascia is opened and left open in order to relieve the pressure.

Fascial Hernia

Some patients with shin splint symptoms are found to have a muscle herniation through the fascia of the compartment. This is usually a small defect through which some muscle tissue is pushed, especially during exercise when the muscle is engorged. The circulation through the herniated tissue may be impaired and result in ischemic pain. The defect may be congenital or traumatic in nature and is usually found in the distal part of the lower leg. The treatment of a painful hernia is surgical whereby the small hernia is enlarged into a full compartment release. This can alleviate the ischemic changes in a small herniation.

Differential Diagnosis of Lower Leg Pain

Acute Pain

✗ Muscle strain (tennis leg)
✗ Muscle contusion
✗ Achilles tendon rupture
✗ Acute compartment syndrome

Chronic Pain

✗ Achilles tendinitis or tendinosis
✗ Traction periostitis
✗ Stress fracture
✗ Chronic compartment syndrome
✗ Muscle herniation

Suggested Readings

Hulkko A, Orava S, Alen M. Stress factures of the lower leg. Scand J Sports Sci 1987;9:1–8.

Letho MUK, Jarvinen MJ. Muscle injuries, the healing process and treatment. Ann Chir Gynaecol 1991;80:102–108.

McKenzie DC, Clement DB, Taunton JE. Running shoes, orthotics and injuries. Sports Med 1985;2:334–347.

Mubarak SJ, Gould RN, Lee YF. The medial tibial stress syndrome. Am J Sports Med 1982;10:201–205.

Puddu G, Scala A, Cerullo G, et al. Achilles tendon injuries. In: Renstrøm PAFH, ed. Clinical practise of sports injury prevention and care. The encyclopedia of sports medicine. Oxford, UK: Blackwell Scientific Publications, 1994:188–216.

Wallensten R, Eriksson E. Intramuscular pressures in the exercise induced lower leg pain. Int J Sports Med 1984;5:31–35.

CHAPTER 14

Ankle and Foot Injuries

Lisa T. DeGnore

More than half of all sports-related injuries occur in the lower extremity. Of these, as many as 30% involve the foot and ankle. The majority of these injuries are to the soft tissue of the foot and ankle, with fractures accounting for only about 5% to 10%. Soft tissue problems include acute and chronic or overuse-type injuries. In this chapter, we will examine foot and ankle anatomy as well as acute and chronic injuries.

In evaluating foot and ankle injury epidemiology, there are both extrinsic and intrinsic factors. In a study reported in 1988, Garrick and Requa found that of 12,681 athletic injuries seen over a 5-year period at a busy sports medicine clinic, 25% involved the foot and ankle. They divided their population into 19 different sports including dance, running, gymnastics, skiing, skating, and all types of ball activities. Running had the highest rate of total injuries to the foot and ankle, with tennis second. Different sports had varying potential for injury to the ankle alone (basketball), to the foot alone (hiking and walking), or to both (modern dance). Some sports such as swimming had a low level of injury to both. Activities that involved cutting, twisting, running, jumping, or uneven terrain had high levels of injury. Thus the type of sports activity is an extrinsic factor in injuries to the foot and ankle.

Other extrinsic factors are shoes, playing surface, coaching, and training methods. Shoes play an important role in foot and ankle injury. The shoe should fit well and be appropriate for the sport. It should also have the correct interface with the playing surface. For example, basketball shoes are designed with rubber treads that prevent slipping on the smooth floor of the court, while football shoes are designed to dig into turf for added traction. The shoe, however, can also play a role in injury. This can be illustrated by the basketball player who falls over a planted foot that "sticks" to the court and inverts the ankle, or the football player who has a hyperextension injury to his great toe in the flexible turf shoe. Shoes may have to be modified for players with foot deformity or who have had previous injury. A pronated foot will benefit from an orthotic insert in the shoe and a player with a previous "turf toe" injury will need a stiffer-toed shoe in order to return to play.

Training and coaching practices can also play a role in injury. The data regarding stretching and conditioning are not always clear as to the exact program necessary to prevent injury, but coaches and trainers should be encouraged to promote regular sessions of stretching and strengthening exercise before sport participation. Moreover, the proper strengthening and range-of-motion program after injury will help players return to their sport. Trainers and coaches can also help players by having reasonable expectations about a player's ability to return to play.

Factors intrinsic to the players affect their risk of foot and ankle injury. These include flexibility, conditioning, and range of motion. Flexibility and range of motion are inherited traits that can be somewhat affected by exercise. For example, with years of intense training, a ballet dancer may develop increased flexibility in his or her feet and ankles. And while this hypermobility may enhance a dancer's ability to perform, it may place him or her at increased risk of either acute or chronic injury. Certainly a regular program of stretching and conditioning exercises before, during, and after the sports season will help decrease injury and may help earlier return to play after injury.

Anatomy

The bones that make up the ankle joint are the tibia, fibula, and talus (Fig. 14.1). This joint acts like a hinge joint, allowing only dorsiflexion and plantar flexion. The medial and lateral stability of the ankle is provided by the deltoid ligament and lateral ligament complex, respectively. The deltoid is one large fan-shaped ligament that originates from the medial malleolus of the tibia. The lateral complex consists of three separate ligaments: the anterior talofibular ligament, the calcaneofibular ligament, and the posterior talofibular

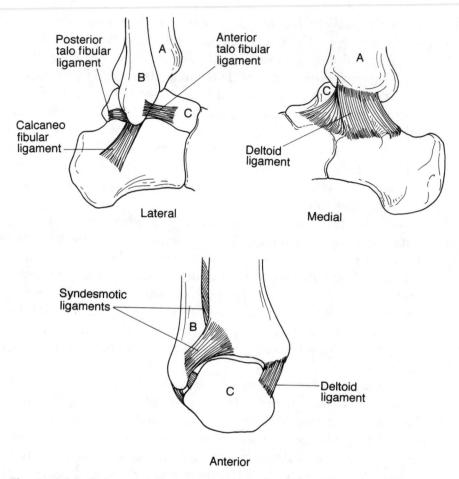

Figure 14.1 *Bones and ligaments of the ankle joint with tibia (A), fibula (B), and talus (C).*

ligament. They originate from the lateral malleolus of the fibula. The tibia and fibula are stabilized together by the syndesmotic ligaments. The hindfoot consists of the talus and calcaneus (Fig. 14.2). The joint between them is often called the subtalar joint. This joint provides the side-to-side motion (inversion and eversion) of the hindfoot. Five additional tarsal bones make up the midfoot. The combined joints between the tarsal and metatarsal bones are called Lisfranc's joints. The five metatarsals connect through the metatarsophalangeal joint with the phalanges of the toes.

The longitudinal arch of the foot is formed by the bones on the medial side of the foot. The navicular bone serves as the keystone at the top of the arch. The ligaments that connect each of the bones support the arch. Additional structures that provide support are the muscle-tendon units of the foot and the plantar fascia. The plantar fascia is a tight fibrous band that originates from the calcaneus and runs to structures in the forefoot (see Fig. 14.2).

The muscles that power the foot and ankle are largely found in the lower leg (Fig. 14.3). Extensor muscles include the extensor hallucis longus attaching to the big toe, the extensor digitorum longus to the lesser toes, and the tibialis anterior muscle to the area of the first tarsometatarsal joint. Ankle and foot flexor muscles include the gastrocnemius-soleus muscle attaching to the calcaneus, the tibialis posterior to the navicular, and the peroneal to the lesser metatarsals. The tibialis posterior and tibialis anterior muscles can also turn in or invert the foot through the subtalar joint. The peroneal muscles can turn out or evert the foot. Similar to the hand, the foot also has small intrinsic muscles within it that contribute to toe movement.

The nerve supply of the foot is largely provided by the peroneal and posterior tibial nerves. The branches of the peroneal nerve provide sensation to the top or dorsum of the foot, whereas the sensation of the bottom or plantar aspect is provided by the posterior tibial nerve.

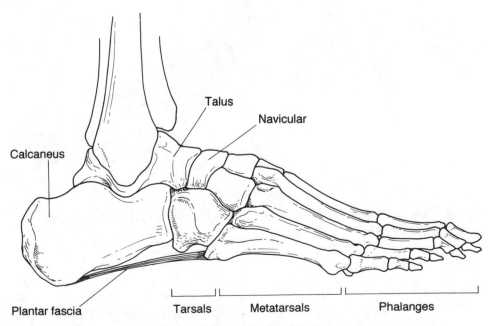

Figure 14.2 *Bones of the foot with the plantar fascia.*

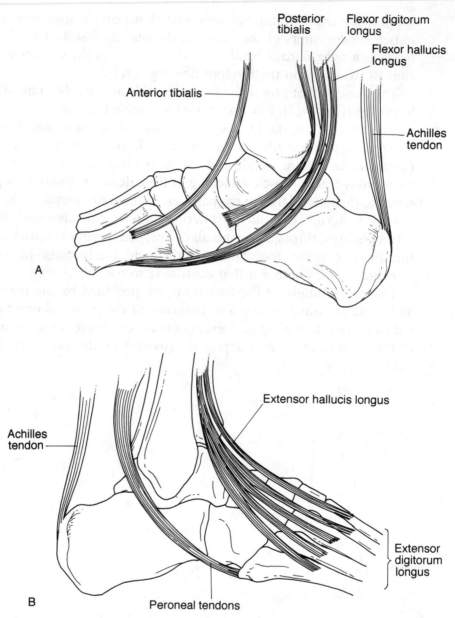

Figure 14.3 *Muscle-tendon units of the medial (A) and lateral (B) aspect of foot and ankle.*

Acute Ankle Injuries

A sudden twist or turn of the ankle is a common cause of acute ankle injuries. The vast majority of these injuries will be ligament injuries or ankle sprains. This section will discuss the different types of sprains in more detail.

Lateral Ligament Sprains

The inversion ankle sprain is one of the most common sports injuries. It occurs in many disciplines, with high frequency among runners and ball players and low frequency among swimmers. The injury commonly occurs during cutting maneuvers or on uneven ground. Foot position, weight, and momentum influence the extent of injury. Greater force will result in a more severe injury. For example, a 200-pound runner whose foot inverts in a pothole will most likely suffer a greater injury than a 130-pound walker who trips on uneven pavement. Excessive force and momentum may result in a fracture rather than a sprain.

The lateral ankle ligament complex consists of the anterior talofibular, calcaneofibular, and posterior talofibular ligaments (see Fig. 14.1). Injury usually begins in the anterior talofibular ligament and progresses posteriorly. Ankle sprains may be graded by the number of ligaments involved (Table 14.1). Grade I injuries involve the anterior talofibular ligament; grade II, the anterior talofibular and the calcaneofibular ligaments; and grade III, the anterior talofibular, calcaneofibular, and posterior talofibular ligaments. A careful physical examination will enable the physician to determine the extent of injury.

Evaluation

When a patient is seen within 24 to 48 hours after the acute injury, the individual ligaments involved in the sprain will be discernible by their local tenderness. Later, diffuse swelling and ecchymosis make the examination more difficult. The examination should begin with observation of the extent of swelling and ecchymosis. In a mild ankle sprain, these will be concentrated over the anterior part of the lateral ligament complex. More severe injuries or those evaluated in the

Table 14.1 Lateral ligaments

SEVERITY	ANTERIOR TALOFIBULAR	CALCANEOFIBULAR	POSTERIOR TALOFIBULAR
Grade I	+	−	−
Grade II	+	+	−
Grade III	+	+	+

Sprains of the lateral ligament complex of the ankle can be graded based on the extent of injury. The ligaments involved will be tender to direct palpation.

subacute setting will have more extensive swelling and discoloration. The examination should progress to evaluation of range of motion and neurovascular assessment. Dorsiflexion, plantar flexion, inversion, and eversion should all be carefully compared with the normal ankle. The examiner should then carefully palpate all bony and ligamentous structures. Point tenderness directly over a ligament strongly indicates a sprain, whereas tenderness directly over the bone, such as the lateral malleolus, should be considered a fracture until proved otherwise. The examiner can also determine the degree of instability as a result of the injury. The anterior drawer test should be performed to assess the stability of the ankle. This is performed with one hand stabilizing the distal tibia while the testing hand places an anterior force on the hindfoot (Fig. 14.4). The patient should be as relaxed as possible during this test to prevent muscle spasms from affecting the assessment. It may have to be repeated when the patient's acute pain has resolved. The drawer test should be evaluated for the distance the talus moves anteriorly in the mortise and the presence or absence of a firm endpoint. The normal ankle should be evaluated for a baseline. Translation of 2 to 3 mm more than on the normal side or lack of a firm endpoint suggests instability. This patient may have recurrent injuries and may ultimately require stabilization.

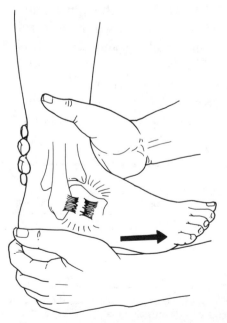

Figure 14.4 *Anterior drawer test of the ankle for a tear of the anterior talofibular ligament.*

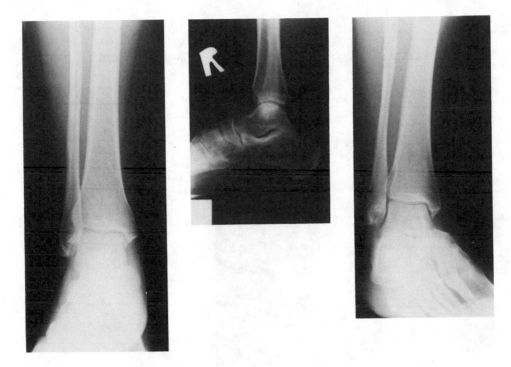

Figure 14.5 *Anteroposterior (A), lateral (B), and mortise (C) views of the normal ankle.*

Three x-ray views of the ankle (anteroposterior, lateral, and mortise) should be obtained for a complete examination, in particular when there is tenderness over the bone. The vast majority of these radiographs will be normal (Fig. 14.5) or show small avulsion fractures of the malleoli. However, the lateral malleolus or lateral process of the talus may be fractured in some patients and can be missed without x-rays (Fig. 14.6).

Treatment

The classic treatment of rest, ice, compression, and elevation (RICE) is essential in the first 24 to 48 hours after injury. Anti-inflammatory medications are important adjuncts for pain relief and their possible anti-inflammatory effect. Subsequently, patients should be instructed in a range-of-motion program that progresses to gait training and strengthening. Patients should be encouraged to ambulate early and may benefit from the use of an ankle corset or brace. Use of several noninvasive modalities such as cryotherapy and ultrasound may be beneficial if they are readily available. Physical therapists and sports

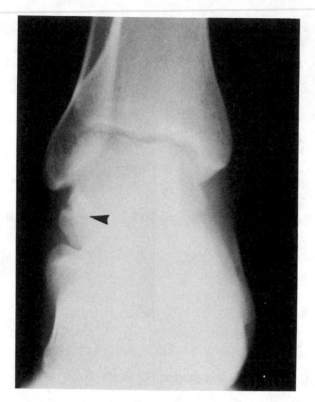

Figure 14.6 *Lateral process fracture following a twisting injury to the ankle.*

trainers can be important team participants in returning high-demand athletes to the playing field or weekend joggers to work. An intensive strengthening program of the lower leg should be initiated as soon as pain permits. This should be supervised in the first week, and players should be given careful instruction in a home program. Prolonged immobilization such as a cast has not been shown to be particularly helpful and may cause significant muscle atrophy and joint stiffness.

Medial Ligament Sprains

Injuries to the deltoid, the medial ligament complex of the ankle, are much less common than lateral ligament injuries. The deltoid is one of the strongest ligaments in the lower leg, and considerable force is required to tear it. A deltoid tear may be accompanied by a distal fibular fracture or a tear of the syndesmotic ligaments. The injury occurs during forced eversion or external rotation of the ankle.

Evaluation

The patient's ankle should again be observed for areas of swelling and ecchymosis, which may be extensive. The patient will be tender distal to the medial malleolus, directly over the deltoid ligament, and not on the malleolus itself. Careful attention should be paid to palpating the other structures of the ankle and foot to find any accompanying injuries. Range of motion, neurovascular status, and stability should be evaluated. The function of the posterior tibial tendon should be assessed because of its proximity to the injury and its potential involvement. This can be done by testing inversion strength while palpating the tendon. Decreased inversion strength indicates a posterior tibial tendon injury.

As discussed above, deltoid injuries are more frequently accompanied by fractures owing to the large forces involved. Three x-ray views of the ankle are necessary for complete evaluation. If there is physical evidence of injury to the foot, anteroposterior and oblique views of the foot should be included in the examination. The mortise view of the ankle should be carefully evaluated for symmetry of both the ankle joint and the syndesmosis. The clear space on all sides of the talus should vary less than 2 mm, and the syndesmosis clear space distance should be 6 mm or less (Fig. 14.7).

Treatment

The treatment for an isolated deltoid sprain is similar to that for a lateral sprain. These patients should be informed that their recovery may be longer owing to the severity of the injury.

Fractures or syndesmotic disruptions that accompany a deltoid tear should be evaluated and treated surgically if necessary.

Injuries to the Ankle Syndesmosis

The exact incidence of injuries to the syndesmotic ligaments of the ankle is not known. They occur in severe external rotation injuries to the ankle. If the force is moderate, the anterior tibiofibular ligament is ruptured, while greater forces lead to disruption of the remainder of the syndesmotic ligaments or interosseous membrane. This can occur, as described previously, in a player who rotates on a planted foot (Fig. 14.8).

Evaluation

The patient with a syndesmotic injury will be tender over the anterior tibiofibular ligaments and proximally over the interosseous membrane between tibia and fibula. The patient may be tender over the deltoid and over the proximal fibula if a fracture has occurred. The proximal extent of tenderness on the leg indicates the proximal extent of the tear. Swelling and ecchymosis are usually extensive, and the

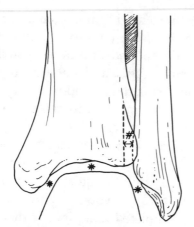

Figure 14.7 *The space between the talus on all sides (*) should vary less than 2 mm and the syndesmosis space (#) should be less than 6 mm.*

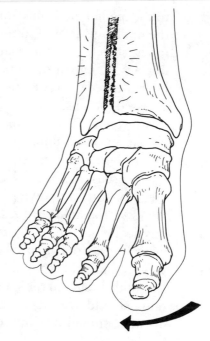

Figure 14.8 *Mechanism of injury for a syndesmosis tear.*

patient will often be unable to bear weight. A careful neurovascular and motor examination is needed to evaluate accompanying injuries. Moreover, the branches of the superficial peroneal nerve cross the ankle near the syndesmosis and may be injured with a sprain.

As with deltoid injuries, a careful examination of joint symmetry is indicated. If a patient has tenderness over the proximal fibula, x-rays should be obtained to look for fractures. The tibiofibular clear space should be measured 1 cm proximal to the ankle joint and should be less than 6 mm (see Fig. 14.7). If there is any uncertainty in measuring this distance, the normal ankle may be x-rayed for comparison. Stress views are obtained to evaluate instability if the syndesmotic distance is not widened but a severe injury is suspected. These are performed with lateral pressure on the foot against a stabilized tibia.

Treatment

If these injuries show no widening of the tibia and fibula on radiography of the syndesmosis and are stable on stress views, they may be treated as a lateral ankle sprain. However, the recovery, in general, is prolonged, and the athlete may not return to play as early as expected. If instability is demonstrated on stress views, the injury may require long leg casting or surgical fixation. An athlete and his or her coach or trainer should be counseled on the potentially prolonged recovery period (6–12 weeks).

Peroneal Tendon Injury

Acute anterior dislocation of the peroneal tendons is a rare injury, but it is more common than acute ruptures. Dislocation occurs with forced dorsiflexion of the inverted foot and contraction of the peroneal muscles. This may occur in skiers during turns or falls if the tips of the skis dig into the snow. The soft tissue injury involves a tear of the peroneal retinaculum that normally holds the tendon in the groove behind the fibula. This allows the tendons to dislocate anterior to the fibula. They frequently snap back into their normal position. If missed initially, subsequent recurrent dislocations of the tendon can occur with minimal trauma. The clue to making the correct diagnosis for recurrent dislocations is the patient's history of a "snapping" feeling and the physical findings of tenderness and swelling along the posterior fibula.

Evaluation

Observation of the injured ankle will show swelling and ecchymosis posterior to the fibula. Tenderness will be present along the posterior border of the fibula. The entire ankle and foot should be examined to evaluate any associated injuries. Neurovascular status, stability, and range of motion should also be evaluated. Motor strength of the peroneal muscles should be tested and may result in pain at the site of injury and a snapping or dislocation of the tendons. This will be most evident when the patient attempts to evert an inverted foot against resistance.

A complete series of ankle x-rays should be obtained. Occasionally an avulsion of the peroneal retinaculum occurs with a thin fragment of fibula.

Treatment

Treatment of the acute dislocation usually involves 4 to 6 weeks in a non-weight-bearing cast. In the past, taping has been advocated, but a high rate of recurrence has been associated with this method. Some authors have discussed surgical repair of the acute injury in the high-performance athlete, but this is controversial. In general, chronic dislocations are treated operatively by a variety of methods.

Ankle Fractures

If x-ray evaluation reveals a fracture line that enters the ankle joint, referral to an orthopedist is generally necessary. Bony small-avulsion chip fractures at the tip of the malleoli can be treated as ankle sprains. The remainder should be carefully evaluated for displacement of the fractures. Surgical reduction with internal fixation is generally necessary for displaced ankle fractures as the risk of posttraumatic arthritis is quite high when an anatomic reduction is not obtained.

Acute Foot Injuries

The foot is exposed to both direct and indirect trauma. Direct trauma usually involves being stepped on by another athlete. Indirect trauma can occur as result of twisting or bending in spite of the protection that is offered by most shoes. This section will discuss the most common acute foot injuries.

Tarsometatarsal Joint or Midfoot Sprain

The tarsometatarsal or Lisfranc's joints are surrounded by extensive soft tissue attachments and form a transverse arch. The plantar ligaments in particular are very strong and provide support to the longitudinal and transverse arch of the foot. Bony stability is provided by the base of the second metatarsal, which "keys" into the row of tarsal bones. This bone acts as the keystone in the center of the transverse arch. Significant force is required to disrupt these joints, and an injury usually involves fractures or fracture and dislocation rather than sprains.

The mechanism of injury involved is one of direct dorsal-to-plantar loading or axial loading combined with twisting. For example, Lisfranc's joints can be injured when a concrete block falls on a construction worker's foot or when a football player falls on another player's planted, plantar-flexed heel. Most athletic injuries to Lisfranc's joint occur during football or soccer, but they also can occur in skiing, horseback riding, and running. In horseback riding, for example, the injury can occur when the rider's foot is trapped in the stirrup after a fall. These injuries involve considerable force, and even simple sprains (without displacement or fracture) may cause long-term stiffness and pain in the foot and may prevent a return to athletics. The exact cause of the persistent pain is unclear, but it may be due to the injury to joint cartilage.

Evaluation

Injuries that result in deformity of the midfoot with fractures or dislocation are readily diagnosed. However, injuries that involve partial ligament tears or those with a spontaneous reduction of a dislocation are more easily missed. Patients with a sprain of Lisfranc's joints will have midfoot swelling and will be tender over the dorsal ligaments of the joints involved. They will have pain in the midfoot when standing on the toes and may be unable to ambulate.

Neurovascular and motor function should be carefully examined because the dorsalis pedis artery and deep peroneal nerve lie directly over the medial Lisfranc's joint and may be injured. In dislocations, tendons may be entrapped in the joint space. In severe dislocations or crush injuries, a compartment syndrome may develop and severely compromise circulation. A compartment syndrome is caused by swelling within a closed tissue compartment of the limb. There are closed tissue compartments in the foot just as in the forearm and the leg. Compartment syndrome should be suspected in a foot with tense, firm swelling, decreased sensation globally, decreased capillary refill, and pain with passive motion of the toes. A late sign is a decreased pulse. This requires prompt surgical decompression to improve blood flow to the toes.

In evaluating any foot injury, three x-ray views must be obtained: anteroposterior, lateral, and oblique (usually internal). Occasionally, an external oblique view may be added to examine complex dislocation. On the anteroposterior view, the first tarsometatarsal-cuneiform joint should be aligned along its lateral border with the base of the second metatarsal (Fig. 14.9). This space should be symmetric, and if there is any question of its being widened, a standing film (stress view) or a normal foot comparison view should be obtained. On the oblique film the medial border of the fourth metatarsal should clearly be aligned with the cuboid.

Treatment

Fractures, fracture-dislocations, and compartment syndromes require prompt surgical attention. Although there is some debate, most authors now recommend open reduction and internal fixation of dislocations and fracture-dislocations. Decompression of a compartment syndrome of the foot requires multiple incisions to open all of the small tissue compartments.

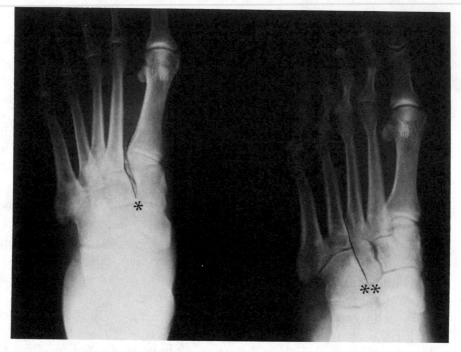

Figure 14.9 *Normal alignment of Lisfranc's joints at the second (*) and fourth metatarsals (**).*

In the more subtle, nondisplaced sprains or partial ligament disruption, use of a non-weight-bearing cast for 6 weeks is advocated, followed by 3 to 6 months of orthotic support. After casting, range-of-motion and strengthening exercises are instituted. Athletes should have full, painless range of motion and no pain with ambulation before returning to their sport. Those with severe injuries may be unable to return to a preinjury level of play owing to chronic pain and stiffness.

Turf Toe

The great toe is a commonly injured digit in athletes. The exact incidence of injury to the toe is unknown, but it is more common among football players and most common when football is played on artificial turf. Hyperdorsiflexion injury to the great toe (the most common mechanism of injury) was described as "turf toe" by Bowers and Martin in 1976. They felt that the injury occurred as a result of players wearing flexible shoes and playing on an unyielding surface (artificial turf). This injury can also occur in soccer players and in aerobic dancers who often land on their dorsiflexed toes. The injury occurs when the toe is forced into dorsiflexion with an axial load (Fig. 14.10). Depending on the position of the foot, a varus or, more commonly, valgus force may be applied with dorsiflexion, which determines the extent of lateral or medial injury to the joint. The dorsiflexion component of this force injures the plantar structures of the joint. These include the plantar plate, the flexor tendons, and the two sesamoid bones within the tendons. The most commonly torn structure is the plantar plate, which avulses from the neck of the metatarsal.

Turf toe injuries have been classified by Clanton (Table 14.2). A grade I injury involves a stretch injury of the plantar capsule. A grade II injury involves a partial tear, and a grade III injury involves a

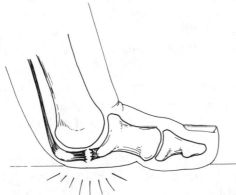

Figure 14.10 *Mechanism of injury for a turf toe.*

Table 14.2 Acute sprains of the first metatarsophalangeal joints

	LIGAMENTS	SYMPTOMS	RANGE OF MOTION	TREATMENT
Grade I	Stretch injury	Mild-moderate	Full	Stiff shoe, taping
Grade II	Partial tear	Moderate-severe	Decreased	1–2 weeks out of play, stiff shoe, taping
Grade III	Complete tear, possible fracture	Severe, unable to weight bear	Markedly decreased	Crutches 2–4 days, 3–6 weeks out of play, stiff shoe, taping

Turf toe injuries are graded by the extent of injury, and treatment is instituted accordingly.

complete tear with or without a fracture of the sesamoids or separation of a bipartite sesamoid.

Soft tissue injuries to the lesser toes are less commonly reported, but even less is known about their exact incidence. The most common mechanism is also a dorsiflexion injury, and the plantar plate is the most commonly torn structure.

Evaluation

The physical examination should include close observation of the foot for swelling, ecchymosis, range of motion, neurovascular evaluation, and careful palpation of tendon structures. Players with a grade I injury will have mild to moderate tenderness over the plantar structures. They will have mild, localized swelling of the joint, and range of motion is usually preserved. They will be able to ambulate with mild discomfort. Players with a grade II injury will have more marked tenderness, swelling that most likely extends into the midfoot, ecchymosis, and decreased range of motion. They may be able to ambulate (with pain), but they will be unable to participate in their sport. With a grade III injury, the player will have severe swelling, ecchymosis, tenderness, and markedly decreased range of motion. Frequently the athlete will be unable to ambulate. If a varus or valgus force has occurred in any of these injuries, the medial or lateral joint capsule will be tender.

Injuries to the lesser toes will cause similar signs and symptoms in the affected toe. Often the injured toe will have a sausage-like appearance.

Patients with more than mild symptoms should have an x-ray. Three views of the forefoot (anteroposterior, lateral, and oblique) should be obtained. They should be carefully examined for avulsion fractures, phalangeal fractures, and sesamoid injuries. If separation of a bipartite sesamoid bone is suspected, the normal foot may be x-rayed for comparison.

Treatment

Treatment is summarized in Table 14.2. Players with a grade I injury may return to playing when comfortable in a stiffer shoe with taping of the toe. The stiff shoe may incorporate a steel plate in the sole of the forefoot, or the player can be custom-fitted with a rigid orthotic. Ice and elevation are important in providing immediate comfort and controlling swelling. A grade II injury will restrict a player's participation in sports. It is important to convince the player and the coach that failure to allow sufficient time for healing may prolong recovery significantly and may predispose the player to chronic injury. These players should be kept out of athletics until their range of motion returns to normal and they are comfortable running in a stiffened shoe. They need early ice, elevation, and taping of the toe. In general, symptoms and motion improve in 7 to 14 days. A grade III injury will probably prevent participation in sports for 3 to 6 weeks. These athletes usually need crutches for ambulation until the most acute symptoms improve. They require strict rest, ice, and elevation and a compressive bandage. When the acute pain and swelling resolve, range-of-motion exercises are started. They may ambulate in a stiff shoe when comfortable, and they may resume play when range of motion is full and tenderness has resolved. Players who return too early have shown a tendency toward chronic injury and disability.

Injuries to the lesser toes are usually treated more simply. The toe should be buddy-taped to an adjacent toe, and sports may be resumed in a stiff shoe when the player is comfortable. The player should be counseled that an injured small toe may remain tender and swollen for more than 8 weeks after injury. Fractures that are nondisplaced or those in which the toe is clinically straight may be treated similarly.

Foot Fractures

Fracture of the tarsal bones can lead to serious posttraumatic problems if not treated correctly. Virtually all tarsal fractures should be evaluated by a specialist.

Metatarsal fractures are more common but fortunately often heal well without serious sequelae. Most metatarsal fractures can be treated with a cast or a stiff-soled shoe and heal in 4 to 5 weeks. The only exception is the fifth metatarsal shaft fracture, which not infrequently goes on to a nonunion.

Phalanx fractures of the toes are also common and heal with minimal intervention. Buddy-taping to the adjacent toe and a stiff-soled shoe can often allow continued activities.

Chronic Foot and Ankle Injuries

The foot and ankle are subjected to large, repetitive loads in virtually every sport. This can lead to chronic injury, particularly in the soft tissues. This last section will discuss the most common chronic injuries of the foot and ankle.

Chronic Ankle Instability

Repeated acute ankle sprains can lead to permanently stretched and deficient ankle ligaments if each acute sprain did not result in complete healing of the injury. Once the ligaments are deficient, the athlete will notice that minimal twists and turns can result in "giving way" of the ankle. This is not uncommon following multiple lateral ligament sprains.

Evaluation

The history is usually significant for multiple turning-in or inversion sprains occurring with increasing frequency. Physical examination can reveal some tenderness over the lateral ligaments if such an episode of giving way occurred recently. Some instability may be noticed on the anterior drawer test of the talus. However, x-rays while the ankle is forced into inversion (stress views) can only determine the actual degree of instability. Comparison stress views of the normal side are important because there is a wide, natural variety in ankle laxity.

Treatment

Most athletes with chronic ankle instability can be managed without surgery. Peroneal muscle strengthening is an important part of the treatment. As evertors they may be able to prevent "turning in" of the ankle if they are strong and contract at the right time. Ankle taping or a lace-up brace have been shown to improve ankle stability during practice or play. This can be reinforced by using high-top athletic shoes. If nonoperative measures are unsuccessful in controlling the instability, surgery can be considered. This restores much of the stability by tightening the existing but lax ligaments or reinforcing them with a graft obtained from local tendons.

Plantar Fasciitis

With each step the body weight is placed upon the longitudinal arch of the foot resulting in a tendency of the foot to roll onto the inside (pronation) and flatten. One of the structures that resists this motion is the plantar fascia. Excessive repetitive impact as well as aging can lead to injury to the plantar fascia. In the vast majority of cases this will occur at its origin from the calcaneus (see Fig. 14.2). Breakdown in this area is called plantar fasciitis.

Evaluation

The athlete usually complains of heel pain that gradually developed. Initially the pain is most severe after a period of rest such as upon arising in the morning. Later the pain also becomes disabling during sports activities. Physical examination reveals tenderness at the origin of the plantar fascia on the calcaneus, usually on the medial side. Flexible flat feet and tight heel cords are also often found.

X-rays often will reveal a spur at the origin of the plantar fascia. This heel spur is merely a reflection of the response of the bone to the traction and irritation by the plantar fascia and not the cause of pain by itself.

Treatment

The initial approach follows the guidelines for chronic overuse injuries in general. Relative rest, nonsteroidal anti-inflammatory medication, and icing are used. This can be reinforced by gentle stretching exercises of both the plantar fascia and the Achilles tendon. Soft heel cups or orthotics can redistribute the stress of impact and help unload the injured area. Recovery, even with this approach, is often slow. In recalcitrant cases, a local corticosteroid injection can be tried. Extreme care should be taken not to inject the fatty heel pad. Steroid atrophy of the heel pad can lead to intractable chronic heel pain. Occasionally a surgical release of the plantar fascia is needed to allow resolution of the symptoms.

Tendinitis

Similar to other parts of the musculoskeletal system, the foot and ankle tendons can develop chronic irritation. This occurs in particular as a response to repetitive use. In the foot the posterior tibialis tendon is particularly prone to this problem. It results in chronic pain over the course of the tendon, occasionally accompanied by localized swelling. In severe cases the tendon can go on to rupture, which often results in an increased flat foot deformity. Treatment of posterior tibial tendinitis is by relative rest, anti-inflammatory medication, and custom-molded shoe inserts or orthotics.

Stress Fractures

Several bones in the foot are susceptible to developing chronic stress fractures. The navicular and lesser metatarsal are known to be common sites for stress fractures. They usually develop in running athletes during training periods of increased intensity or duration. X-rays and occasionally bone scans are needed to visualize the fracture. Treatment may involve casting and limitation of weight bearing. Occasionally surgery is needed to stimulate healing of stress fractures.

Differential Diagnosis of Ankle and Foot Pain

Ankle Pain

Acute Pain

- ✗ Ankle sprain
- ✗ Ankle fracture
- ✗ Peroneal tendon dislocation
- ✗ Acute episode of chronic instability

Chronic Pain

- ✗ Chronic instability
- ✗ Recurrent peroneal tendon dislocations
- ✗ Tendinitis
- ✗ Arthritis

Foot Pain

Acute Pain

- ✗ Midfoot sprain
- ✗ Fracture
- ✗ Dislocation

Chronic Pain

- ✗ Plantar fasciitis
- ✗ Tendinitis
- ✗ Stress fracture
- ✗ Arthritis

Suggested Readings

Bowers KD, Martin RB. Turf-toe: a shoe-surface related football injury. Med Sci Sports Exerc 1976;8:82–83.

Clanton TO, Butler JE, Eggert A. Injuries to the metatarsalphalangeal joints in athletes. Foot Ankle 1986;7:162–176.

Delee JC, Drez D, eds. Foot and ankle. In: Orthopaedic sports medicine. Phila-
    delphia: WB Saunders, 1994:1632–2034.
Garrick JG, Requa RC. The epidemiology of foot and ankle injury in sports. Clin
    Sports Med 1988;7:29–36.
Harper MC, Keller TS. A radiographic evaluation of the tibiofibular syndesmo-
    sis. Foot Ankle 1989;10:156–160.
Mann RA, ed. Surgery of the foot. St. Louis: CV Mosby, 1986.
Stover CN, Bryan DR. Traumatic dislocation of the peroneal tendons. Am J Surg
    1962;103:180–186.

Index